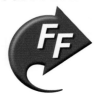

Fast Facts

Fast Facts:
Sexually Transmitted
Infections

Second edition

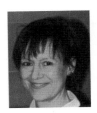

Anne Edwards MD FRCP
Consultant Physician
Honorary Senior Clinical Lecturer
Genitourinary Medicine
The Radcliffe Infirmary, Oxford, UK

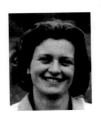

Jackie Sherrard MD FRCP
Consultant Physician
Genitourinary Medicine
The Radcliffe Infirmary, Oxford, UK

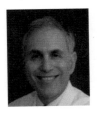

Jonathan Zer
Professor of Mec
Chief, Infectious
Johns Hopkins Bayview Me...
Baltimore, USA

Declaration of Independence
This book is as balanced and as practical as we can make it.
Ideas for improvement are always welcome:
feedback@fastfacts.com

✝ HEALTH PRESS

Fast Facts: Sexually Transmitted Infections
First published May 2001
Second edition February 2007

Text © 2007 Anne Edwards, Jackie Sherrard, Jonathan Zenilman
© 2007 in this edition Health Press Limited
Health Press Limited, Elizabeth House, Queen Street, Abingdon,
Oxford OX14 3LN, UK
Tel: +44 (0)1235 523233
Fax: +44 (0)1235 523238

Book orders can be placed by telephone or via the website.
For regional distributors or to order via the website, please go to:
www.fastfacts.com
For telephone orders, please call 01752 202301 (UK), +44 1752 202301 (Europe),
1 800 247 6553 (USA, toll free) or +1 419 281 1802 (Americas).

Fast Facts is a trademark of Health Press Limited.

A CIP record for this title is available from the British Library.

ISBN 978-1-903734-95-7

Edwards, A (Anne)
Fast Facts: Sexually Transmitted Infections/
Anne Edwards, Jackie Sherrard, Jonathan Zenilman

The cover shows a colored scanning electron micrograph of
Neisseria gonorrhoeae bacteria (round) on a human epithelial cell.
Credit: Science Photo Library.

Medical illustrations by Dee McLean, London, UK.
Typesetting and page layout by Zed, Oxford, UK.
Printed by Fine Print (Services) Ltd, Oxford, UK.

Text printed with vegetable inks on biodegradable and
recyclable paper manufactured from sustainable forests.

444 001
Low emissions
during production

Low
chlorine

Sustainable
forests

Glossary of abbreviations

AIDS: acquired immune deficiency syndrome

CPPS: chronic pelvic pain syndrome

DGM: dark ground microscopy

FTA-ABS: fluorescent treponemal antibody-absorbed [test]

GUD: genital ulcer disease

GUM: genitourinary medicine

HAART: highly active antiretroviral treatment

HBeAg: hepatitis B 'e' antigen

HBsAg: hepatitis B surface 's' antigen

HBV: hepatitis B virus

HCV: hepatitis C virus

HIV: human immunodeficiency virus

HPV: human papillomavirus

HSV: herpes simplex virus

HTLV: human T-cell lymphotropic virus

Ig: immunoglobulin

LGV: lymphogranuloma venereum

MSU: midstream urine

NAAT: nucleic acid amplification test

NSU: non-specific urethritis

PCR: polymerase chain reaction

PID: pelvic inflammatory disease

PPV: positive predictive value

RPR: rapid plasma reagin

RT-PCR: reverse transcriptase polymerase chain reaction

STI: sexually transmitted infection

UTI: urinary tract infection

VDRL: venereal disease research laboratory

Introduction

Sexually transmitted infections (STIs), particularly human immunodeficiency virus (HIV) infection, are an important cause of morbidity and mortality worldwide, and are responsible for the loss of many productive years. They have a disproportionate impact on adolescents and young adults.

In developed countries, the incidence of most viral and bacterial STIs is increasing. The World Health Organization estimated that in 1999 there were 340 million cases of selected curable STIs (gonorrhea, *Chlamydia* infection, syphilis, chancroid and trichomoniasis), 90% occurring in resource-poor countries. Among the sexually active population, the prevalence of herpes simplex type 2 infection and of sexually transmitted human papillomavirus infection is estimated to be 20–40% and 30–60%, respectively. These rates are higher in developing countries. Since 1998 there has been an upsurge of STIs in homosexual men, a trend that has profound implications for the epidemiology of STIs and HIV infection.

The annual cost of STIs is estimated at US$7.18 billion in the USA, and that of treating the short-term effects of STIs at £700 million in the UK. Two STIs – gonorrhea and chancroid – no longer respond reliably to readily available and inexpensive antimicrobials and, increasingly, expensive third-generation cephalosporins and fluoroquinolones are required to treat these two diseases, causing particular problems in resource-poor areas.

STIs are important cofactors in the sexual transmission of HIV. In addition, the treatment of a number of STIs has become more challenging in immunocompromised individuals with HIV infection. Every family physician now encounters patients with STIs. We hope that *Fast Facts: Sexually Transmitted Infections* will provide a useful summary of current thinking on the diagnosis and effective management of these wide-ranging infections.

Treatment guidelines

The treatment guidelines presented in each chapter are adapted from the UK guidelines for the management of STIs. The US recommendations (2006) have been added where these differ from the UK guidelines. Full details of the US recommendations can be found in the Centers for Disease Control and Prevention publication *Clinical prevention guidance. Sexually transmitted diseases treatment guidelines 2006* (*MMWR Recomm Rep* 2006;55:1–94; www.guideline.gov).

Each patient should be assessed individually for history of drug allergy, pregnancy risk and other medication that may result in interactions. All treatment is oral unless otherwise stated. All tetracycline-based antibiotics are contraindicated in pregnancy.

Epidemiology

It is well established that a number of pathogens are transmitted sexually (Table 1.1). Several other common syndromes cause genital tract symptoms, but sexual transmission is not established, or is less important; these include bacterial vaginosis (an ecological disturbance of vaginal flora) and genital candidiasis.

Diagnoses of most sexually transmitted infections (STIs) have increased in recent years. Figures 1.1 and 1.2 show annual incidences in the UK and the USA, respectively. In the USA, the Centers for Disease Control and Prevention estimate that over 15 million STIs are diagnosed each year. The impact of STIs and their associated complications (Table 1.2) on public health is considerable.

Treatment and control

Successful control of STIs depends on:

- early diagnosis – screening programs are often required as many STIs are asymptomatic
- effective treatment (for curable infections), with oral and single-dose regimens wherever possible, ideally free for the patient
- contact tracing – referral and treatment of sexual partners
- education – behavioral risk reduction and prevention of transmission
- counseling and voluntary testing for human immunodeficiency virus (HIV) – this should be an integral part of any STI control program, as HIV is mostly transmitted sexually, and other STIs facilitate HIV transmission (on both a biological and a behavioral basis).

STIs are frequently asymptomatic, particularly in women. People with asymptomatic infection may not perceive themselves to be at risk of infection and may not access healthcare services. When asymptomatic infection is detected by screening, identified infected individuals may be less likely to comply with treatment or partner referral recommendations.

TABLE 1.1

Sexually transmitted pathogens

Viral pathogens

- Herpes simplex virus (genital herpes): HSV 1 and HSV 2
- Human immunodeficiency virus (HIV)
- Human papillomavirus (genital warts)
- Hepatitis B virus
- Human herpesvirus-8 (Kaposi's sarcoma)
- Human T-cell lymphotropic viruses: types 1 and 2 (HTLV1 & 2)
- Cytomegalovirus
- Hepatitis C virus – sexual transmission occurs occasionally (< 5% cases)
- Molluscum contagiosum – caused by a member of the Poxviridae family

Ectoparasites

(transmission occurs through close contact, sexual intercourse is not required)

- *Phthirus pubis* (pubic lice)
- *Sarcoptes scabiei* (scabies)

Bacterial pathogens

- *Chlamydia trachomatis*
- *Neisseria gonorrhoeae* (gonorrhea)
- *Treponema pallidum* (syphilis)
- Genital mycoplasmas (including *Mycoplasma genitalium*)
- *Haemophilus ducreyi* (chancroid)
- *Klebsiella granulomatis* (donovanosis)
- Overgrowth of predominantly anaerobic organisms (e.g. *Gardnerella vaginalis*, *Orevotella* spp., *Mycoplasma hominis*, *Mobiluncus* spp.) in the vagina is characteristic of bacterial vaginosis*

Protozoa

- Intestinal protozoa (amebiasis, giardiasis)
- *Trichomonas vaginalis*

Fungi

- *Candida* spp. (may be passed from female to male partners)

*Bacterial vaginosis is seen almost exclusively in women who have been sexually active but the relevance of sexual transmission is not clear.

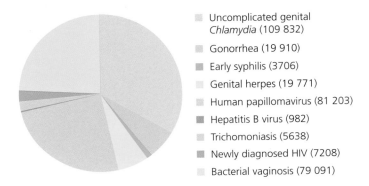

Figure 1.1 Infections diagnosed at genitourinary medicine clinics in the UK in 2005.

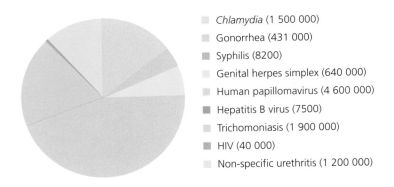

Figure 1.2 The estimated annual incidence of the most common STIs in the USA.

STIs frequently coexist, so the presence of one should lead to screening for others. For each infected individual identified, there is always at least one other infected individual, who may not be receiving treatment. Notification and treatment of sexual partners reduces the risk of reinfection in an individual and improves public health by limiting

9

TABLE 1.2

Complications associated with sexually transmitted infections

Female reproductive tract

- Pelvic inflammatory disease
- Chronic pelvic pain
- Ectopic pregnancy
- Tubal infertility

Male reproductive tract

- Epididymitis
- Prostatitis

Perinatal

- Miscarriage/stillbirth
- Vertical transmission and neonatal disease
- Premature rupture of membranes
- Chorioamnionitis
- Low birth weight

Others

- Anogenital cancers
- Structural damage/scarring
- Systemic complications, e.g. disseminated gonococcal infection, reactive seronegative arthritis (formerly known as Reiter's syndrome)
- Increased transmission of human immunodeficiency virus

spread in the community, although the best strategy for achieving this (by the patient or by the health service) may depend on a number of factors.

Strategies. In the UK, genitourinary medicine departments remain the cornerstone of any strategy aimed at treating and preventing STIs. These services are open access, free at the point of delivery and confidential. Clinics are equipped with on-site diagnostic facilities, usually involving microscopy, allowing a preliminary diagnosis to be made at the initial attendance. In the USA, about 50% of public health departments offer STI services of varying accessibility and quality, usually at no cost or with 'sliding-scale' fees based on ability to pay. STI screening, especially for *Chlamydia*, is increasingly being seen as a quality assurance measure.

Key points – epidemiology and control

- A number of bacteria, viruses and parasites are transmitted sexually. Bacterial vaginosis and genital candidiasis affect the genital tract but are not considered to be sexually transmitted infections (STIs).
- Many STIs are asymptomatic, particularly in women.
- Control of STIs depends on early diagnosis through screening programs; effective, ideally free, treatment; referral and treatment of sexual partners; education about behavioral risk reduction; and prevention of transmission.
- Counseling and voluntary testing for human immunodeficiency virus (HIV) should be an integral part of any STI control program, as HIV is mostly transmitted sexually and other STIs facilitate HIV transmission.
- STIs frequently coexist, so the presence of one should lead to screening for others.

Approach to the patient

Risk assessment

The many recognized risk factors and markers for STIs are summarized in Tables 2.1 and 2.2. Assessment of a patient's risk factors can aid diagnosis, and can also improve the cost-effectiveness of screening by enabling physicians to select appropriate tests. Risk assessment may involve a self-administered questionnaire or a face-to-face interview. To be effective, an interview should be frank, open and non-judgmental. STI risk assessment should be integrated with a general health risk assessment consistent with the specific clinical setting, such as primary care or family planning, and ideally should form part of the general

TABLE 2.1

Risk factors for sexually transmitted infections

- Multiple partners (two or more in the last year)
- Concurrent partners
- Recent partner change (in past 3 months)
- Non-use of barrier protection
- Infection in partner
- Other sexually transmitted infection
- Younger age (particularly aged ≤ 25 years)

TABLE 2.2

Risk markers for sexually transmitted infections

- Residence in or travel to a high-prevalence area
- Low socioeconomic status
- Not married
- Previous infection

preventive medical assessment (i.e. an assessment should be performed for all patients, not just those suspected of having an STI). In the USA, *Chlamydia* screening is now recommended for all women under 25 years of age who are sexually active.

Evidence suggestive of an STI. When assessing risk, the possibility of an STI should be considered:

- if any risk factor or marker is present (see Tables 2.1 and 2.2)
- if new genital symptoms have developed, particularly after a change of sexual partner
- following sexual assault
- in any sexually active teenager
- if there are signs/symptoms of any of the classic STI syndromes (see later chapters)
- if pelvic pain or other symptoms of pelvic inflammatory disease are present
- if the patient reports dyspareunia
- if epididymitis is seen in a man under 35 years of age
- if genital warts are present.

In some situations, epidemiological concerns should heighten suspicion. People living in or visiting highly endemic areas are at increased risk of STIs, as are military personnel on deployment, and travelers, who may have contact with multiple new sex partners, including commercial sex workers.

Referral

Patients with any of the following symptoms should be considered for referral to a genitourinary medicine (GUM) or STI specialist for diagnosis and management:

- unusual/recalcitrant vaginal discharge
- pelvic pain or lower abdominal pain not requiring emergency admission
- urethral discharge/dysuria
- undiagnosed genital ulcers
- undiagnosed genital rash.

Children

STIs in neonates and infants usually result from perinatally acquired infection; perinatally acquired genital warts may present well into childhood. Although perinatal acquisition is possible in older children, some infections, such as gonorrhea and chlamydial infection, strongly suggest the possibility of sexual abuse. In such cases, further investigations by the appropriate authorities are warranted and children should be referred to an appropriate specialist.

Advising a patient with a suspected STI

A patient who may have an STI should be advised to abstain from sexual intercourse until they have been screened and diagnosed and have completed their course of treatment. Their partner(s) will also need to be fully investigated and any treatment completed before sexual activity can be resumed.

Sexual history

A full sexual history is vital for diagnosis and risk assessment (Table 2.3) and allows the physician to provide appropriate and relevant advice for the future. It is important that the physician taking the history is able to make the patient feel comfortable, feels comfortable themselves asking the questions (he or she should have received training in this area) and adopts a non-judgmental approach. The one-to-one interview, carried out with the assurance of confidentiality, is ideally performed in a soundproof room. If this is not possible, patients should be assured that their interviews will not be overheard.

Genital examination

A genital examination should be performed after taking a sexual history. Many STIs cause no symptoms, and it is not uncommon for clinical findings to be at odds with patients' descriptions of their symptoms. Failure to perform a genital examination and/or appropriate tests may result in an incorrect diagnosis. It is particularly important to examine individuals whose symptoms have either failed to respond to, or have recurred following, empirical therapy.

TABLE 2.3

Sexual history

Signs/symptoms: establish the duration and nature

- Discharge – urethral/vaginal/rectal
- Dysuria
- Lumps or bumps – genital/inguinal region
- Cuts or ulcers
- Pain – pelvic, testicular or other genital pain, including dyspareunia

Sexual partner(s), recent and current

- Male/female
- Date of most recent contact
- Duration of relationship
- Presence or absence of symptoms
- Country of origin/history of recent travel

Personal information

- Sexual practices (e.g. genital–genital, orogenital)
- Use of barrier protection
- Drug/alcohol use, particularly at the time of last sexual intercourse (as this is more likely to result in non-use of condoms and thus increase the risk of STI transmission)

- Previous history of STI and diagnosis
- Previous testing for human immunodeficiency virus
- Country of origin/history of recent travel

Drugs

- Current medication
- Vaccinations (e.g. hepatitis B)
- Recent antimicrobials
- Drug allergies

Women

- Date of last menstrual period
- Method of contraception/protection
- Pregnancy risk
- Date of last cervical (Pap) smear
- History of intermenstrual or postcoital bleeding

The examination room should be warm and comfortable. As speculum examinations are recommended for women, a table or couch with stirrups is useful. Good lighting is essential.

The entire genital and perianal area should be inspected in both sexes, and the inguinal nodes palpated. In uncircumcised men, the foreskin should be retracted and the area examined completely. Examination of men should also include inspection of the urethral meatus and palpation of the testes and epididymides. Proctoscopy (anoscopy) is recommended in gay men who practice receptive anal intercourse.

In women, a speculum examination allows inspection of the vagina and cervix. Uterine and adnexal tenderness and masses can be assessed by a bimanual pelvic examination.

The development of highly sensitive urine-based DNA amplification tests, such as the polymerase chain reaction (PCR) has ignited a debate on whether a full examination is required. The authors' opinion is that within a clinical setting, a full genital examination, including, in women, a speculum examination with cervix visualization, is strongly recommended. Where tests are being undertaken as part of a screening program, examination is essential in any patient with symptoms. Increasingly, however, screening is taking place without a speculum examination, for example in venue- and school-based screening.

Further examination

Depending on the symptoms and signs, a more detailed general examination may be necessary. This should include examination of the skin, the mouth for ulcers and, if reactive seronegative arthritis or gonococcal arthritis are possible, the joints.

Tests

The tests that should ideally be included in a basic screening are described in Table 2.4. Other tests may be performed, depending on symptoms, signs and diagnoses in sexual contacts.

Diagnostic microscopy is available in most GUM departments, and the diagnosis is often made while the patient is still in the clinic. This enables treatment to be initiated and contact tracing and counseling to be undertaken at the first visit.

TABLE 2.4
Basic screening tests

Women

- Vaginal samples for wet preparation, pH measurement and Gram stain for trichomoniasis, candidiasis and bacterial vaginosis
- Endocervical, introital and/or urethral samples to test for *Neisseria gonorrhoeae* and *Chlamydia trachomatis* (depends on local diagnostic tests)
- Syphilis serology
- Human immunodeficiency virus (HIV) test (with patient's consent)
- If at risk of gonorrhea, pharyngeal and rectal samples for *N. gonorrhoeae*, and a Gram stain of rectal discharge if symptomatic (proctoscopy is not required)
- Routine herpesvirus serological testing is a matter of debate

Men

- Urethral smear for Gram stain to detect gonococci or increased number of neutrophils, consistent with non-gonococcal urethritis (if available)
- Urethral swab or first-pass urine sample to test for *N. gonorrhoeae* (test dependent)
- Urethral swab or first-pass urine sample for *C. trachomatis* (test dependent)
- Syphilis serology
- HIV test (with patient's consent)
- If at risk of gonorrhea, pharyngeal tests for *N. gonorrhoeae*
- Routine herpesvirus serological testing is a matter of debate

Additional tests for men who have sex with men

- Pharyngeal swab for *N. gonorrhoeae*
- Rectal sample to test for *N. gonorrhoeae* if history of receptive anal intercourse (even with condom use), and a Gram stain of rectal discharge if symptomatic
- Screening for hepatitis B if no history of vaccination

Counseling

The perceived risk of an STI and an actual diagnosis can cause stress and anxiety. However, STIs are rarely life-threatening, and the greatest concerns for patients are the implications for their current sexual partner(s) and their future sex and reproductive lives.

Part of the role of the health professional is to communicate information effectively and accurately in order to reassure the patient and to facilitate contact tracing when necessary. A critical part of the process includes advising patients about preventing re-exposure and reinfection, sometimes referred to as counseling. The following two dictionary definitions encompass most elements of counseling in the context of STIs:

- (a service consisting of) helping people to adjust to or deal with personal problems, etc. by enabling them to discover for themselves the solution to the problems while receiving sympathetic attention from a counselor
- (sometimes) the giving of advice on miscellaneous problems.

General approach. Counseling is usually the final part of the consultation and provides an opportunity to:
- explain about specific diagnoses
- discuss contact tracing where relevant
- give general information about safer sex practices and risk reduction.

Most counseling by health professionals is actually patient education. Research has demonstrated, however, that behavior change (i.e. adopting prevention-oriented behavior, such as consistent condom use) requires time and effort. Modern counseling techniques incorporate factors such as:
- interactivity – working with the patient to understand the context in which risk behavior occurs; this avoids the imposition of preconceived ideas by the counselor and allows the patient to do most of the talking
- identification of realistic goals – patient-centered counseling permits realistic goals to be developed in the context of the individual's race/ethnicity, culture, knowledge and socioeconomic status

- contracting – defining incremental contractual objectives (e.g. 100% condom use with new sexual partners or arranging STI screening every 3 months)
- reinforcement – identifying steps already taken, encouraging continued avoidance of risk behavior and negotiating additional risk-reduction targets.

Adopting intensive counseling techniques clearly requires time and resources, and triage may be necessary. Counseling should include an assessment of technical skills (e.g. instruction on correct use of condoms).

Key concepts in STI counseling. The following key concepts are useful in helping couples to avoid misunderstandings when an STI diagnosis is made.

Latency. Many STIs, particularly the viral infections, display latency. They may be dormant, causing symptoms months, or even years, after initial acquisition. A diagnosis does not, therefore, automatically imply infidelity.

Asymptomatic carriage. Many infected patients will have no symptoms. The diagnosis may be made because a partner acquires an STI and becomes symptomatic, or because an individual decides to have a check-up. For this reason, it may not be possible to determine the duration of infection or to identify the source partner.

Recurrent disease. Contact tracing and treatment of partner(s) for the bacterial STIs are crucial. The most common reason for so-called recurrent infection of a bacterial disease is reinfection from an untreated partner. Some infections, usually the viral STIs, and genital herpes in particular, cause recurrent disease because they cannot be eradicated with existing treatment options. Despite this, for the majority of affected individuals further problems are usually minor and easily managed. This important message is an essential part of patient education, as many misconceptions abound among the general public. For example, most people diagnosed with cold sores (oral herpes) do not react to the news with 'But it's incurable', yet this phrase is a common response to a diagnosis of genital herpes.

Consent for investigations

It is considered good practice to obtain consent for all investigations. In many clinical settings, however, particularly for the diagnosis of treatable and/or non-life-threatening conditions, specific consent need not be sought. In the USA, with the exception of HIV testing, consent is usually implied in the general consent for care that patients are asked to sign. HIV testing requires separate consent, and in some states a specific consent form may be mandated. However, this is a dynamic area and there is a movement towards routine HIV testing and elimination of the separate consent process. In the UK, specific consent for HIV testing should be sought, apart from in some exceptional circumstances (Table 2.5).

Human immunodeficiency virus infection

An initial risk assessment that explores sexual lifestyles, drug usage and World Health Organization pattern II country risk (countries in which spread of HIV is predominantly through heterosexual sex) will determine whether an individual requires full pretest counseling or a pretest discussion. Full counseling is usually reserved for patients at high risk of HIV infection (Table 2.6 and Figure 2.1).

Reasons for HIV testing include:
- patient request
- as part of an evaluation for STIs (full infection screening)
- to identify infected individuals who might benefit from therapeutic intervention (including women planning a pregnancy or who are already pregnant)
- to counsel the high-risk patient in order to reduce the risk of acquisition, or of transmission if already infected
- to provide partner notification for contacts of those who test positive, for the above reasons
- clinical: when HIV infection may be part of the differential diagnosis in a symptomatic patient (see Chapter 11).

Pretest discussion has become simplified in recent years. Most believe that, for low-risk patients, it is reasonable to ensure that the patients understand:

TABLE 2.5

Circumstances in which HIV testing may be undertaken without specific consent*

Circumstance	Guidance
Organ donation from deceased patient	Explain the need to test for HIV to relatives
Post-mortem testing	Where ordered/authorized, test for communicable disease if relevant to investigation into the cause of death
Injury to health worker	If the source patient is unconscious, seek consent to test once consciousness is regained If health worker is seriously injured and there is a risk of HIV infection, take prophylactic action You may test without consent if the patient dies and you have good reason to believe that they may have been infected
Unconscious patient	When testing would be in their immediate clinical interests
Children	When they cannot give or withhold consent, consent should be sought from someone with parental authority
Sexual assault perpetrators	Compulsory testing may be required by some states in the USA (not in the UK)

*Based on guidelines from the UK General Medical Council. In the USA, each state has its own policy, although HIV testing is becoming more routine.

- why they are considered to be at low risk
- the window period – detectable antibodies almost always appear within 3 months from the time of infection
- confidentiality
- the arrangements for giving results.

21

TABLE 2.6

Groups at high risk of HIV infection

- Homosexual/bisexual men and their sexual partner(s) (male/female)
- Intravenous drug users and their sexual partner(s)
- Those who have lived in or visited an area where the main mode of HIV transmission is via heterosexual activities*
- Partners of those who have lived in or visited an area where the main mode of HIV transmission is via heterosexual activities*
- Those at risk from contaminated blood/blood products
- Commercial sex workers
- Heterosexuals who practice unprotected penetrative sex with multiple partners

*World Health Organization pattern II countries.

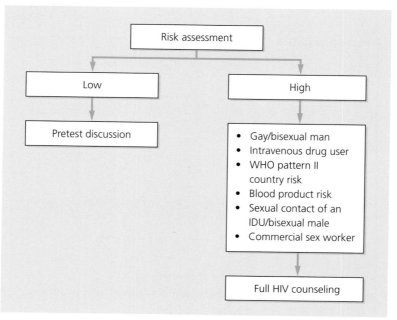

Figure 2.1 HIV testing and the relative risk of certain patient groups. IDU, intravenous drug user; WHO, World Health Organization.

Full counseling. In addition to the areas covered in the pretest discussion, counseling for patients at high risk of HIV infection should include:

- detailed discussion of the implications of a positive result for both the individual and their sexual partner(s)
- an exploration of support networks
- stressing that HIV infection is treatable (though not curable).

This also presents an opportunity to inform patients about risk reduction and safer sex practices.

Patients who present for care who have had high-risk behavior or STI exposure and who have a viral or flu-like illness should be considered at risk for acute HIV syndrome (primary HIV infection).

Before counseling, details of patients' sexual practices should be obtained. For example, whether they:

- use barrier methods of protection
- have a history of anal sex (highest risk), with or without protection, and/or unprotected vaginal intercourse.

If patients use intravenous drugs, try to determine details of related practices, for example, whether they share needles with others.

Giving results

Ideally, all high-risk individuals should be advised of their HIV test result in person. However, most would now agree that low-risk patients can obtain their results without necessarily visiting the clinic.

The positive result. Give the patient the result as quickly and humanely as possible. If the patient has been tested in a non-specialist setting, local HIV services can be contacted in advance of giving the result to facilitate rapid access for repeat testing and for post-test counseling. Most patients, however well prepared, will be distressed. All newly diagnosed patients must be given time with an experienced health professional to consider the implications of the result. They should be provided with written information, including the details of support organizations. When the patient leaves, they should have a clear idea of who they will discuss the result with at this early stage. Optimism is perhaps one of the most important messages: there are many exciting

23

advances in therapy, and most patients will remain healthy for many years. If possible at this visit, or at an early follow-up visit, the patient should have a medical evaluation (including measurement of viral load and CD4 count) either on site or by referral. This facilitates rapid access to expert medical care.

Most patients will be asked to have a repeat or confirmatory HIV test at their referral visit. In addition, newly diagnosed HIV-positive patients will need to think about partner notification, which should also have been considered during the initial counseling session. In the UK, health advisers working in GUM clinics will routinely address these issues. In most US states, HIV infection is now a reportable disease. Unless testing is performed at an anonymous site, case information will be reported to the local health department.

Risk reduction and prevention of STIs

An important element of managing a patient who has an STI or who is at risk of acquiring one is the opportunity to educate about risk reduction. The main risk factors for STI acquisition are described earlier in this chapter (see Table 2.1). Educating patients about minimizing these risk factors, including the consistent use of barrier methods of protection, is most effective in a one-to-one setting. This is, however, an expensive way of undertaking health promotion. Educating adults who work with young people is an important means of cascading information to those most at risk. The goals in sexual-health promotion are to increase attendance and eventually reduce the positive pick-up of infections and their long-term complications in people undergoing screening for STIs.

Vaccinations have been developed for human papillomavirus (HPV) and hepatitis B. These are covered on page 100 and pages 106 and 108, respectively.

Key points – approach to the patient

- Risk assessment by a self-assessment questionnaire or interview aids diagnosis and improves the cost-effectiveness of screening.
- A sexual history and genital examination are important aspects of assessment.
- Counseling involves advising patients about preventing re-exposure and reinfection, particularly by contact tracing and treatment, and is a key part of the consultation.
- Patients considered to be at high risk for HIV infection require full counseling before undergoing an HIV test.
- Patients who test positive for HIV require considerable support from health professionals, and should be referred for specialist care.
- Sexual health promotion – particularly with adults who work with young people – is a key strategy in reducing the incidence of STIs.

Urethritis is a syndrome characterized clinically by dysuria and/or discharge (Figure 3.1) and/or urinary frequency. The symptoms may be intermittent or persistent and of varying severity and chronicity. Urethritis is asymptomatic in 30–40% of men, although examination may reveal objective evidence of discharge (up to 50%).

If specific pathogens such as *Neisseria gonorrhoeae* or *Chlamydia trachomatis* are isolated, the condition is termed gonococcal or chlamydial urethritis, respectively. In the absence of specific pathogens, the terms non-specific urethritis (NSU) or non-gonococcal urethritis are used. NSU can be defined as an inflammation resulting from an as-yet unidentified, and therefore pathogen-negative, infection of the distal urethra.

Nucleic acid amplification tests have established that 30–60% of apparently pathogen-negative NSU is chlamydial (Table 3.1). Other etiologic agents include certain species such as *Mycoplasma genitalium* and *Ureaplasma* species (20–40% of cases altogether). In a typical clinical setting, tests for *Mycoplasma* and *Ureaplasma* species are not carried out routinely. Herpes simplex virus and *Trichomonas vaginalis*

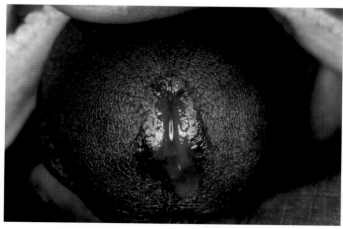

Figure 3.1 Urethral discharge in a man with non-specific urethritis.

TABLE 3.1

Organisms associated with urethritis

Agent	Comment
Neisseria gonorrhoeae	Common
Chlamydia trachomatis	30–60%
Ureaplasma urealyticum	10–20%
Mycoplasma genitalium	10–20%
Pathogen-negative organisms not yet identified	20–40%
Herpes simplex virus	Rare, particularly if no signs
Adenoviruses	Associated with orogenital contact
Trichomonas vaginalis	Rare (possibly more common in developing countries)

are occasionally implicated, and adenoviruses are implicated in some cases, often in association with orogenital contact. In men who have sex with men, enteric organisms may cause urethritis. However, in many cases no pathogens can be identified, despite intensive investigations.

Strictly speaking, urethritis is confined to men. However, it is recognized that women can have urethral chlamydial infection, and that some women have a urethral syndrome, possibly with the same etiology as male NSU. This syndrome is sometimes termed the dysuria–pyuria syndrome, and presents as a urinary tract infection (UTI) that is culture-negative for the typical UTI organisms. In addition, there is a group of probable genital pain syndromes – interstitial cystitis and the urethral syndrome – that mimic urethritis symptomatically and do not appear to have an infectious etiology (Chapter 8). The remainder of this chapter refers to male urethritis only.

Transmission

NSU is predominantly sexually acquired. The causative agent(s) may be transmitted through unprotected genital or orogenital contact. Female contacts are commonly asymptomatic, but run the risk of developing pelvic infection if they remain untreated. Asymptomatic men are more likely to have female partners who present with complicated infection, for obvious reasons.

Investigations

A standard STI screen should be performed (see Table 2.4, page 17). Also consider:

- a urine dipstick test – this may be useful if a UTI is suspected
- culture of a midstream urine (MSU) sample if the urine dipstick test and/or history is suggestive.

Diagnosis

Urethritis is indicated by the finding on a Gram-stained urethral smear, taken at least 2 hours after the last voiding, of five or more leukocytes per high-powered field. In symptomatic men with negative urethral smear tests and cultures, a repeat test on a urethral smear obtained after an overnight urine hold may confirm the diagnosis. The diagnosis of NSU is one of exclusion (Table 3.2). Tests for specific causative pathogens should be negative and there should be no evidence of other localized problems that could explain a urethral inflammatory exudate.

Complications

These include:

- epididymitis
- subfertility
- reactive seronegative arthritis
- chronic pelvic pain syndrome (prostatitis, chronic NSU)/chronic testicular pain syndrome (which may follow an episode of urethritis); see Chapter 8.

Management

First presentation of uncomplicated NSU. Treat any other condition that may be causing an increase in leukocytes (Table 3.2). If no other cause is identified, treat for NSU (Table 3.3). In men with urethritis and

TABLE 3.2

**Causes of increased leukocytes on a urethral smear –
differential diagnoses for urethritis**

Diagnosis	Comments
Balanitis	Any cause
Urethral warts	May bleed
Cystitis	Proximal infection, usually abnormalities on urine dipstick test
Chronic non-bacterial prostatitis	May also have genital pain
Stricture/anatomic abnormality	Usually causes cystitis (i.e. urinary tract infection)

another infection, do a repeat urethral smear at follow-up after completing treatment for the other infection. If the urethritis has persisted, treat as for NSU.

Recurrent or persistent NSU is a common and problematic area, and it is widely recognized that the diagnosis of NSU is unsatisfactory. Gram staining is subject to considerable inter- and intra-observer variation. After a first episode, men may complain of minor persistent symptoms that do not necessarily indicate continuing infection. Against this background, it is difficult to interpret follow-up smear tests and it is unwise to base the decision to give more antibiotics purely on a repeated Gram stain. In general, it is important not to perform follow-up tests on men with uncomplicated, pathogen-negative infection who are either better or improving and have complied fully with the recommended treatment regimen. Most patients will respond to reassurance.

Recurrent NSU is more common in men with non-chlamydial NSU and with infections where *M. genitalium* or *U. urealyticum* are implicated. An approach to the management of men with persistent symptoms (i.e. lasting longer than 4 weeks after completing a course of antibiotics) is outlined in Figure 3.2.

TABLE 3.3

Treatment guidelines for non-specific genital infections (including non-specific urethritis) and asymptomatic contacts of patients with non-specific urethritis, pelvic inflammatory disease or epididymitis

Recommended regimens

- Doxycycline, 100 mg twice daily for 7 days
- Azithromycin, 1 g as a single dose

Alternative regimens

- Erythromycin, 500 mg four times daily for 7 days, or twice daily for 14 days
- Chlortetracycline hydrochloride–tetracycline hydrochloride–demeclocycline hydrochloride, 300 mg twice daily for 7 days
- Ofloxacin, 200 mg twice daily for 7 days, or 400 mg once daily for 7 days
- Tetracycline, 500 mg four times daily for 7 days

Regimen in pregnancy

- Erythromycin, 500 mg four times daily for 7 days, or twice daily for 14 days

Contact treatment

- Use recommended regimens

Contact tracing/partner notification

Current and recent partners (6 months is a reasonable cut-off) of men with NSU should be screened and treated, even if tests are negative (Table 3.3). Sexual intercourse should be avoided until both partners have completed antibiotic therapy (this should be stressed even if condom use is proposed).

Prevention

Reliable and consistent use of condoms should prevent most
infections.

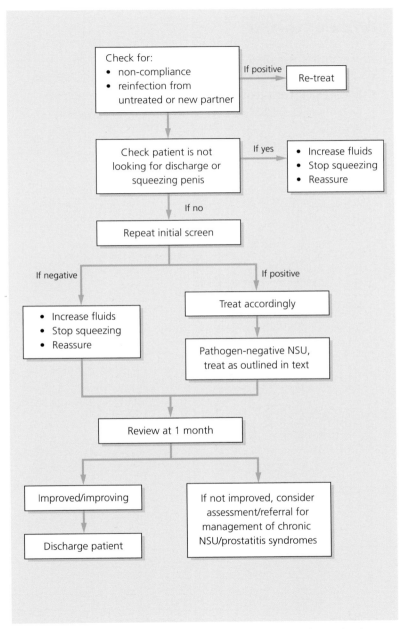

Figure 3.2 Management of persistent/recurrent non-specific urethritis (NSU).

Key points – urethritis

- Urethritis is asymptomatic in 30–40% of men.
- Urethritis is commonly, but not exclusively, caused by *Chlamydia*.
- Recurrent or persistent symptoms in adequately treated men who are not at risk of reinfection are unlikely to have an infective etiology.

4 Vaginal discharge

Vaginal discharge is common and is often not pathological. Normal discharge ranges in appearance from mucoid to opaque, and in quantity from minimal to copious, and the quality and quantity of discharge may vary over the menstrual cycle and over a woman's lifetime.

Most women are aware of a change from their normal pattern; it is therefore not surprising that a spontaneous complaint of abnormal vaginal discharge has good positive predictive value for the detection of pathology. Leading questions and the investigation of asymptomatic discharge are less helpful and may result in asymptomatic women becoming concerned.

Associated vulvovaginal symptoms may provide clues to the etiology. For example, in some women an underlying vulval disorder may be relevant; a careful history and examination should distinguish this patient group (see Chapter 5).

Recent studies have confirmed that most infectious discharge is caused by vaginal pathogens (Table 4.1). Purely cervical infections (e.g. gonorrhea or chlamydial infection) are rarely responsible for vaginal discharge, which, in this setting, is usually due to concomitant vaginal infection, such as bacterial vaginosis (Figure 4.1) or *Candida* vulvovaginitis (Figure 4.2). Women may not appreciate this difference between vaginal and cervical infection, and the cause of discharge needs to be resolved by physical examination.

Assessment and investigation

A history and examination should be undertaken (see Chapter 2). The assessment should routinely include a drug history (with particular emphasis on antibiotic use), and any associated vulvovaginal symptoms should be noted (Table 4.2). Women with poorly controlled diabetes may present with troublesome vulvovaginal candidiasis. The vulval skin should be inspected carefully to exclude any underlying dermatoses (see Chapter 5). If vaginal discharge is observed during an examination, it is important to establish whether the discharge is usual for the

TABLE 4.1

Common causes of vaginal discharge

Epidemiology	Comments
Bacterial vaginosis	

• Most common cause of abnormal discharge in women of childbearing age
• Prevalence increased:
  – in African/Afro-Caribbean women
  – with intrauterine contraceptive devices
  – with recent partner change
  – in women with STIs (probably)
	• Sexually associated but not an STI
	• pH < 4.5 almost always excludes the diagnosis

Candida spp.	
• In 20% of women there is normal carriage • Increased colonization in pregnancy (30–40%) • Uncontrolled diabetes • HIV infection • High-dose estrogens	• Premenarche and postmenopausal women rarely have problems with *Candida* • Routine cultures are unnecessary • Self-limiting vulvovaginal symptoms are common and are often not related to *Candida* (50% of women who self-treat probably do not have candidiasis) • Recurrent vaginal candidiasis is not a marker for HIV infection
Trichomonas vaginalis	
• Common in resource-poor countries, but 5 million cases occur annually in the USA • This is an STI • Asymptomatic in 10–50% of cases	• Increased risk of adverse pregnancy outcome • Cytology is not reliable for diagnosis, which should be confirmed with a microbiological test

HIV, human immunodeficiency virus.

34

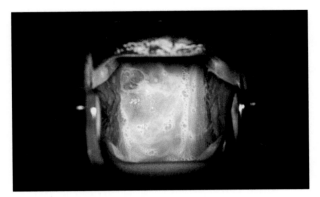

Figure 4.1 Typical discharge of bacterial vaginosis.

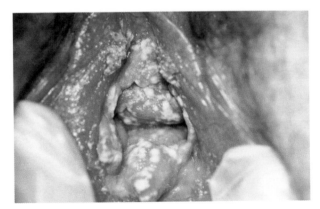

Figure 4.2 *Candida* vulvovaginitis.

woman, as there is little point in investigating asymptomatic discharge unless it is clearly pathological. The characteristics of the discharge may provide a clue about the causative agent (Table 4.2). A Gram-stained slide can indicate 'normality' and is useful in managing pathogen-negative vaginal discharge because it allows the physician to reinforce a diagnosis of physiological discharge. Some women who are peri- or postmenopausal may present with a watery discharge that is pathogen-negative and may be associated with superficial dyspareunia and erythema. Treatment with topical estrogens nightly for 2 weeks, alternate nights for 4 weeks and then twice weekly for 6 weeks can be highly effective.

35

TABLE 4.2

Diagnosis of vaginal discharge

Features/clues	Diagnosis
Candida spp.	
• Itch	• Gram stain
• 'Cottage cheese' discharge	• Culture
• Vulvitis (sometimes)	
Bacterial vaginosis	
• Malodor, worse with intercourse	• Gram stain/wet preparation
• Not usually associated with vulvovaginitis	• pH likely > 4.5
	• Whiff test
Trichomonas vaginalis	
• Vulvovaginitis	• Wet preparation
• Strawberry cervix	• Laboratory test
• Asymptomatic in 50–80%	
Neisseria gonorrhoeae	
• Rare cause; women with gonorrhea commonly have bacterial vaginosis (up to 50%)	• Exclude other causes
Chlamydia trachomatis	
• Rare cause of discharge (asymptomatic in 70–80%)	• Exclude other causes
• Occasional mucopurulent cervicitis	
Primary/first-episode herpes simplex virus infection	
• Frank vulvovaginitis, cervicitis and genital/cervical ulceration	• Investigate if discharge persists after treatment
• Responds to antiviral therapy (antibiotics not indicated)	
• Recurrent infection rarely causes discharge unless another infection is present	

(CONTINUED)

TABLE 4.2 (CONTINUED)
Diagnosis of vaginal discharge

Foreign body
- Anaerobic/malodorous
- Discharge resolves with removal of foreign body
- Antibiotics not usually required

- Investigate if discharge persists after removal

Ectropion/erosion
- Pathogen-negative discharge often attributed but evidence is slender
- Rarely improved by cryocautery (not recommended)

- Exclude infection

Polyp
- Rare cause of discharge

- Exclude infection

Cervical cancer
- Rare cause, but should be clinically obvious

- Colposcopy and biopsy

Estrogen deficiency/menopause
- Watery discharge
- Vulval erythema

- Exclude infection
- Topical estrogens

Treatment
Refer to the appropriate chapter if a pathogen is identified. Treatment guidelines for candidiasis and penile candidiasis are given in Table 4.3, and for peri- and postmenopausal discharge on page 35. Vaginal commensals such as streptococcal species rarely cause discharge, and antibiotics are often incorrectly prescribed as treatment.

It is important to stress normality to the patient if no treatable cause of discharge is found.

Pregnancy
Yeast carriage increases in pregnancy, as do the rates of symptomatic candidiasis, but there are no associated complications. Both bacterial

TABLE 4.3

Treatment guidelines for candidiasis

Vulvovaginal infection

Recommended regimens

- Imidazole pessary, single dose
- Nystatin, two pessaries daily for 14 days

US guidelines

- Nystatin, one 100 000 unit vaginal tablet for 14 days
- Butoconazole 2% cream, 5 g intravaginally for 3 days or single application of sustained-release product
- Clotrimazole 1% cream, 5 g intravaginally for 7–14 days
- Clotrimazole, 100 mg vaginal tablet for 7 days, or two tablets for 3 days
- Miconazole 2% cream, 5 g intravaginally for 7 days
- Miconazole vaginal suppository, one 100 mg or 1200 mg suppository for 7 days or one 200 mg suppository for 3 days
- Tioconazole 6.5% ointment, 5 g intravaginally in a single application
- Terconazole 0.4% cream, 5 g intravaginally for 7 days
- Terconazole 0.8% cream, 5 g intravaginally for 3 days
- Terconazole, one 80 mg vaginal suppository for 3 days

Alternative regimens

- Fluconazole, 150 mg as a single dose (first line in the USA except if pregnancy risk)

Regimen in pregnancy

- Treat according to recommended regimens
- Oral therapy is contraindicated
- Longer courses may be necessary

(CONTINUED)

TABLE 4.3 (CONTINUED)
Treatment guidelines for candidiasis

Contact tracing

- Not usually required, as candidiasis is not transmitted sexually
- Consider for women who have recurrent infection as male partner may have balanitis (see Chapter 5).

Penile infection

Recommended regimen

- Imidazole 1% cream, applied two or three times daily until signs resolve
- Any of the other cream preparations described above

Contact tracing

- None required

vaginosis and infection with *Trichomonas vaginalis* may be associated with an increased risk of adverse pregnancy outcome (see Chapters 9 and 12, respectively).

Recurrent candidiasis

Some women experience repeated episodes of candidiasis. A careful history and microbiological confirmation of the diagnosis are important. Recurrent candidiasis is usually defined as at least four episodes each year, with a minimum of two positive culture tests. Undiagnosed diabetes should be excluded and in the majority of cases will not be found.

Once recurrent candidiasis is confirmed, a 3–6-month trial of suppressive therapy can be tried. One regimen is 1 week's treatment with an oral agent (fluconazole or itraconazole) as induction, followed by fortnightly maintenance with either a single-dose topical agent or 1-day systemic therapy. This can be discontinued after 3–6 months to determine subsequent patterns of infection. However, up to 60% of cases relapse in the 6 months after cessation of treatment. If there is relapse between treatments, the maintenance treatment can be taken weekly.

Occasional cases may be caused by non-albicans species, such as *C. glabrata*. Speciation and sensitivity testing may be useful in women who appear not to respond to therapy, as the non-albicans types can be less sensitive to conventional antifungal therapy.

Key points – vaginal discharge

- Asymptomatic vaginal discharge does not need investigation.
- Physiological discharge is variable and may not be treatable (e.g. cryotherapy for ectropion in such settings is not evidence-based and may not have any effect).
- Sexually transmitted pathogens such as *Chlamydia trachomatis* and *Gonorrhoeae* species rarely cause vaginal discharge.
- Vaginal commensals such as *Streptococcus* species rarely cause discharge, and antibiotics are often incorrectly prescribed as treatment.

5 Genital dermatoses, vulvitis and balanitis

Inflammation of the genitals is a frequent cause of distress and psychosexual morbidity in both men and women. In most cases the underlying cause is not serious, but patients are frequently poorly managed and conditions are treated partially or inadequately.

The external genital tract may be affected by a variety of inflammatory skin and infectious disorders that are not sexually transmitted. Healthcare providers may overlook common (and uncommon) skin disorders in the differential diagnosis of genital dermatoses. Such disorders include allergic and inflammatory disorders such as genital psoriasis, seborrheic dermatitis, atopic eczema and allergic contact dermatitis; the genital dermatoses, such as lichen sclerosus and lichen planus; premalignant and malignant conditions; systemic and rheumatological diseases such as psoriasis, Behçet's syndrome and postinfection arthritis, and common skin infections including cellulitis and fungal dermatitis. The sections below therefore include diseases that are not sexually transmitted.

Vulvitis

Vulvitis is inflammation of the vulva and may be associated with itch/soreness, erythema and superficial (entry) dyspareunia. Vulval symptoms have a range of infective and dermatologic causes (Table 5.1). Some infective causes of vaginal discharge also cause vulvitis (see Chapter 4).

Assessment, investigation and management. There is overlap with women presenting with vaginal discharge; see Chapter 4 for initial assessment. The history should determine the pattern of symptoms, for example intermittent episodes that are self-limiting and shortlived may suggest recurrent vulval herpes (see Chapter 10). Where there is no evidence of infection, the most frequent causes of vulval symptoms are dermatologic, ranging from dry/sensitive skin, lichen simplex and vulval eczema to

TABLE 5.1

Non-infective causes of vulvovaginal symptoms (negative microbiology)

Features	Diagnosis and management
Allergy/irritants	
• Symptoms may be associated with use of a causative agent • May be past history of sensitivity	• Avoidance • Allergy patch testing may help
Dermatoses	
• Genital site may be first presentation, but patient may have past history of or current eczema, psoriasis or seborrheic dermatitis	• Skin examination ± biopsy • Moisturizing agents ± topical corticosteroids
Lichen sclerosus	
• Vulval/perianal (not vaginal) skin involved	• Biopsy • Refer to specialist
Lichen planus	
• May involve vagina and oral mucosa	• Biopsy
Vulval intraepithelial neoplasia	
• May have history of genital warts or cervical intraepithelial neoplasia • Causes irritation	• Biopsy • Refer to specialist
Estrogen deficiency	
• Peri-/postmenopausal women (may occur despite systemic hormone replacement)	• Try topical estrogen therapy
Vulval pain syndrome (vulvodynia/vulvar vestibulitis)	

• Usually normal vulval appearance, but symptoms may include:
  – burning/chronic vulval pain
  – superficial dispareunia
	• Exclude other pathology
	• Refer to specialist

specific genital dermatoses, of which lichen sclerosus and lichen planus are the most frequent. Estrogen deficiency may be the cause in peri- and postmenopausal women (see Chapter 4). If there is no skin abnormality, a vulval pain syndrome should be considered (see Chapter 8). Where skin abnormality is present, a vulval biopsy should be considered. Use of moderate-to-potent topical corticosteroids may alter the histology and should be avoided until a definite diagnosis has been made.

Simple first-line approaches to management include allergen and soap avoidance, and the use of soap substitutes and moisturizers such as aqueous cream. Women who have clear vulval abnormalities and/or whose symptoms do not respond to simple measures should be referred for an expert opinion.

Balanitis

Balanitis is inflammation of the glans of the penis, and can involve the foreskin in uncircumcised men. It may be associated with erythema, irritation, soreness, exudate (mimicking urethral discharge) and dysuria. The presenting features provide clues to the underlying diagnosis (Table 5.2).

Assessment, investigation and management. A full history and examination (see Chapter 2) focusing on the sexual risk, duration and pattern of symptoms will provide clues to etiology. Some acute STIs, including gonorrhea and herpes, may be associated with balanitis. Dermatologic causes are often relatively longstanding and may have a relapsing and remitting course. Where there is abnormality, consider simple management including avoidance of allergens and soap, and the use of soap substitutes and moisturizers such as aqueous cream, but refer patients with persistent changes. Where the skin is normal but does not respond to simple treatments, the cause may be a chronic pelvic pain syndrome (see Chapter 8).

TABLE 5.2

Causes of balanitis

Infection/condition	Features
Infectious	
Candida spp.	• Itch • Erythema, edema, boggy mucosa • Punctate or margin to rash • Female partner may have yeast carriage or symptomatic candidiasis
Anaerobic balanitis	• Exudative • Malodorous • Uncommon in circumcised men • Partner not usually relevant
Streptococcal (rare)	• Erythematous • Painful
Herpes	• See Chapter 10
Non-infectious	
Allergy/irritant (common)	• Skin type • History of allergy/sensitivity
Circinate balanitis	• Associated with reactive seronegative arthritis
Plasma cell/Zoon's balanitis	• Occurs only in uncircumcised men • Distinct erythematous lesion • Benign
Penile intraepithelial neoplasia Erythroplasia of Queyrat Bowen's disease Bowenoid papulosis	• Distinct erythematous patches • Premalignant (~5% risk of malignancy)
Lichen planus	• Papular/marginal/annular rash • May have oral lesions
Lichen sclerosus	• Skin disorder (preferentially affects genital skin) • White patches involving foreskin/glans/urethra • Tightening foreskin • Meatal stenosis
Penile cancer (rare)	• Ulcerated/fissured/hypertrophic lesion (rare)

Diagnosis	Management
• Microscopy and culture • Exclude undiagnosed diabetes	Topical antifungal agents ± partner treatment
• Microscopy and culture	Usually responds to salt washes and improved hygiene
• Culture	Salt washes ± systemic antibiotics
• Clinical	Avoid potential allergens, including implicated creams, ointments, soaps and laundry detergents
• Usually clinical • Biopsy is non-specific	Topical corticosteroid for 3–4 weeks
• Clinical and biopsy	Topical corticosteroid
• Biopsy	Destructive or excisional treatment
• Clinical and biopsy	Topical corticosteroid
• Clinical and biopsy	Potent topical corticosteroid
• Biopsy	Refer to urologist

Key points – genital dermatoses, vulvitis and balanitis

- The key issues when taking a history are the duration of symptoms, presence or absence of itch and rash, whether the problem relapses and remits, treatments already tried and level of sexual risk.
- Examination is essential to identify or exclude definite abnormality; where a dermatological diagnosis is suspected, the whole skin should be examined.
- The patient should be seen when most symptomatic.
- Improvement may be seen with simple approaches such as avoidance of soap and allergens, and use of moisturizers.
- Moderate-to-potent topical corticosteroids should not be used without a diagnosis.

6 / Genital ulcer disease

Genital ulcers, defined as epithelial defects in the skin or mucosa of the genitalia, are a common symptom in both sexes. The common STI causes of genital ulcers are shown in Table 6.1. The etiology of ulcers varies across the world; for example, chancroid is common in sub-Saharan Africa, whereas genital herpes is the most common cause in Europe.

Differential diagnosis

The differential diagnoses (other than those conditions listed above) are wide ranging and include a number of sexually transmitted pathogens. Relatively common causes include:

- trauma – mechanical or chemical self-inflicted or excessive attempts at cleaning
- pyogenic (e.g. ruptured furuncle or infected hair follicle)
- allergy – fixed drug eruption, Stevens–Johnson syndrome.

Uncommon and rare causes include:

- ulceration secondary to parasitic infections (e.g. pediculosis and scabies)
- tuberculosis
- Behçet's disease/aphthosis
- premalignant conditions
- carcinoma
- herpes (varicella) zoster (shingles) limited to genital dermatomes.

Conditions that may be diagnosed incorrectly as ulcers when the epithelium is still intact are:

- severe candidal balanitis/vulvitis
- circinate balanitis in reactive seronegative arthritis
- balanitis associated with Vincent's organisms
- plasma cell (Zoon's) balanitis
- irritant dermatoses
- fixed drug eruption.

TABLE 6.1

Common sexually transmitted infections that cause genital ulcer disease (GUD)

	Primary genital herpes	Primary syphilis	Lymphogranuloma venereum	Chancroid	Granuloma inguinale
Distribution	Commonest cause of GUD in UK	GUD may be seen in primary, secondary and, rarely, tertiary syphilis	Endemic in tropics and subtropics	Mainly tropical regions	Mainly tropical regions
Incubation	7–21 days	9–90 days	3–12 days	3–10 days	7–120+ days
Prodrome	Yes	No	No	No	No
Primary lesion	Vesicle	Papule	Vesicle, ulcer or papule Often inconspicuous	Papule	Papule/nodule
Painful	Yes	No	Variable	Yes	No
Number of ulcers	Multiple	Usually solitary	Solitary	Multiple	One or two
Lymphadenopathy	Yes, painful	Bilateral, painless	May suppurate, usually unilateral	Tender, may suppurate, usually unilateral	No, pseudobubo
Time to healing if untreated	10–21 days	Up to 42 days	Few days then bubo develops	Chronic ulcer	Local spread with chronicity

Diagnosis

This can usually be made from the history and examination, with the aid of selective tests. When examining a patient it is important to determine that ulceration is truly present and that the lesion is not simply erythema. When the ulcer is due to an STI, there is often associated inguinal lymphadenopathy. For patients in whom chancroid, lymphogranuloma venereum (LGV) or granuloma inguinale (donovanosis) are highly unlikely from a travel history, the differential diagnosis is between herpes, syphilis and non-STI causes. Be aware of atypical presentation of common disorders. In the UK and USA, tests for herpes from the ulcer should be performed routinely. Type-specific serological tests for herpes simplex virus (HSV) 1 and HSV 2 may have a role, particularly in a patient with recurrent ulceration and repeatedly negative tests for herpes from the ulcer. HSV-2 antibodies are indicative of genital herpes whereas HSV-1 antibodies do not differentiate between genital and oropharyngeal infection (see chapter 10 for more details.) Syphilis serology should be routinely requested.

Investigations where causes other than HSV are possible:

- HSV swab
- STI screen
- syphilis serology; repeat in 2 weeks if necessary and after a month if still no diagnosis
- dark-ground microscopy on at least three different occasions for *Treponema pallidum* (if syphilis is possible)
- consider biopsy if there is a clinical suspicion of carcinoma (especially if the patient is over 50 years old), donovanosis or obscure diagnosis.

If a tropical STI is a possibility, also:

- swab for *Chlamydia trachomatis* using nucleic acid amplification technology (for LGV) or lymph node aspirate and/or paired sera for *Chlamydia* serology (2-week interval)
- specific culture of ulcer material for *Haemophilus ducreyi* (chancroid)
- screen for granuloma inguinale only for patients presenting with unusual forms of ulceration where other diagnoses have been ruled out and a suggestive travel history is obtained.

Management

Management is as for the underlying condition (see relevant pages).
If obvious superinfection and incubating syphilis cannot be excluded,
saline bathing is the first line of management. If antibiotics are felt to be
necessary, doxycycline or penicillins must not be used, as these will
partially treat undiagnosed syphilis.

Key points – genital ulcer disease

- Genital ulcers are a common symptom in both sexes.
- The etiologies of ulcers differ around the world; for example,
  chancroid is very common in sub-Saharan Africa, whereas genital
  herpes is the most common cause in Europe.
- The differential diagnoses are wide-ranging and include a
  number of sexually transmitted pathogens.
- The diagnosis can usually be made from history and examination
  with the aid of selective tests.

---

7 Pelvic inflammatory disease and epididymo-orchitis

Pelvic inflammatory disease

Pelvic inflammation, which may be acute (lasting less than 1 month) or chronic (lasting for longer than 1 month), is usually triggered by a sexually acquired infectious agent (Table 7.1). The condition is thought to occur because the sexually acquired agent – with or without another trigger (e.g. postpartum, insertion of an intrauterine contraceptive device, medical or surgical termination of pregnancy, or other surgical procedures such as dilatation and curettage) – disrupts the normal cervicovaginal defense mechanisms. This allows the STI and/or usually non-pathogenic agents (e.g. enteric organisms, streptococci or anaerobes) access to the normally sterile upper genital tract. Pelvic inflammatory disease (PID), symptomatic or asymptomatic, is thought to occur in 20–30% of untreated gonococcal and chlamydial infections.

PID represents inflammation of the upper genital tract, including endometritis, salpingitis, oophoritis and pelvic peritonitis. It presents on a continuum, ranging from asymptomatic through to symptoms that are mild and intermittent to very severe. Severe infection probably accounts for only 5–10% of all PID cases. Women with silent infection may present with late complications, including tubal infertility or ectopic pregnancy.

Symptoms may include some or all of the following:
- pelvic pain (may be unilateral), constant or intermittent
- deep dyspareunia
- vaginal discharge (usually due to concurrent vaginal infection)
- irregular and/or more painful menses
- intermenstrual/postcoital bleeding
- fever (unusual in mild/chronic PID).

Signs, at least one of which should be present when making a diagnosis of PID, are:
- cervical motion pain (cervical excitation)
- adnexal tenderness (commonly bilateral but may be unilateral)
- elevated temperature (unusual in mild/chronic infection).

TABLE 7.1

Infective agents that cause pelvic inflammatory disease

Infective agent	Comment
Neisseria gonorrhoeae	Up to 30% of patients also have *Chlamydia* infection
Chlamydia trachomatis	Specific tests are often negative – diagnosis is clinical
Anaerobes	
Enteric organisms	
Gardnerella spp. *Haemophilus* spp.	Usually cause damage following infection by *N. gonorrhoeae* or *C. trachomatis*
Streptococci	
Mycoplasma spp.	Possibly implicated
Ureaplasma spp.	
Mycobacterium tuberculosis	Rare cause (important in developing countries)
Salmonella typhi	Rare cause (important in developing countries)
Actinomyces	Rare cause: actinomyces-like organisms may be reported in association with intrauterine contraceptive devices (only rarely associated with pelvic inflammatory disease)

Diagnosis is clinical and is based on the history and clinical findings. Laparoscopy enables external inspection of the uterus and fallopian tubes and is the diagnostic gold standard, despite the fact that it has never been validated. In most settings, however, widespread use of laparoscopy is impractical. Furthermore, laparoscopy does not reliably exclude endometritis and low-grade salpingitis, which may be present without abnormal laparoscopic findings. Laparoscopy is usually reserved for women in whom therapy has failed. Endometrial biopsy may be useful, but is not widely practiced. Negative microbiological tests do not exclude a diagnosis of PID – a point that cannot be overemphasized.

Differential diagnoses include:

- ectopic pregnancy
- irritable bowel syndrome or inflammatory bowel disease
- endometriosis
- appendicitis (some women presenting with apparent appendicitis have pelvic infection)
- rupture, bleeding or torsion of ovarian cysts
- breakthrough bleeding in women taking combined oral contraceptives.

To exclude these conditions, the following investigations should be undertaken:

- full STI screening, including microbiological tests for *Chlamydia trachomatis* and *Neisseria gonorrhoeae* (see Table 2.4, page 17)
- a pregnancy test if appropriate.

A complete blood count is not essential (white cell count, erythrocyte sedimentation rate and C-reactive protein may be raised in acute PID, but changes are unlikely in chronic/late disease).

Management. As a general principle, it is safer to overdiagnose PID and give antibiotics than not to treat. The risk of tubal infertility is approximately 12% with one episode of PID but increases to some 60–75% with three episodes or more. Women thought to be at risk of infection (see Table 2.1, page 12) who are undergoing gynecologic procedures such as insertion of an intrauterine contraceptive device or termination of pregnancy should have routine screening with antibiotic cover. Treatment guidelines are summarized in Table 7.2.

Contact tracing/partner notification. Current and recent partners should be screened for STIs. If tests are negative, they should be treated as for uncomplicated non-specific urethritis/*Chlamydia* infection (see Tables 3.3 and 9.3, pages 30 and 66). A common cause of apparent treatment failure is reinfection by an untreated partner. Reinfection also substantially increases the risk of fertility problems.

Pregnancy. PID is rare in pregnancy; other explanations for lower abdominal pain should be excluded before making a diagnosis of PID in this setting.

TABLE 7.2

Guidelines for outpatient treatment of pelvic inflammatory disease*

Recommended regimens

UK

- Doxycycline, 100 mg twice daily for 2 weeks, plus metronidazole,[‡] 400–500 mg twice daily for 5–14 days
- Ofloxacin,[†] 400 mg twice daily for 2 weeks, plus metronidazole,[‡] 400–500 mg twice daily for 5–14 days

USA

- Levofloxacin,[†] 500 mg orally once daily for 14 days or ofloxacin,[†] 400 mg orally once daily for 14 days, with or without metronidazole,[‡] 500 mg orally twice daily for 14 days

Alternative regimens

UK

- Levofloxacin, 250 mg once daily for 2 weeks, plus metronidazole,[‡] 400–500 mg twice daily for 5–14 days
- Erythromycin, 500 mg three times daily for 14 days, plus metronidazole,[‡] 400–500 mg twice daily for 5–14 days

USA

- Doxycycline 100 mg orally twice daily for 14 days, with or without metronidazole,[‡] 500 mg orally twice daily for 14 days, plus one of the following:
  - ceftriaxone, 250 mg intramuscularly in a single dose
  - cefoxitin, 2 g intramuscularly in a single dose and probenacid, 1 g orally administered concurrently in a single dose
  - other parenteral third-generation cephalosporin (ceftizoxime or cefotaime)

Regimen in pregnancy

- Erythromycin, 500 mg three times daily for 14 days, plus metronidazole,[‡] 400–500 mg twice daily for 5–14 days

(CONTINUED)

TABLE 7.2 (CONTINUED)

Guidelines for outpatient treatment of pelvic inflammatory disease*

Contact treatment
- Treat as non-specific genital infection (see Table 3.3, page 30)

*In areas with a high prevalence of gonorrhea, or if a patient is at risk of gonorrhea, treat for gonorrhea concurrently (see Table 9.4, page 72).
†In some areas of the world, such as the Far East and Pacific Islands, there are high rates of resistance to quinolones and penicillin. The US Centers for Disease Control recommend that patients with gonorrhea acquired in these areas should not be treated with quinolone-based regimens.
‡Metronidazole provides anaerobic coverage; anaerobic organisms are suspected in the etiology of the majority of cases of pelvic inflammatory disease.

Bartholin's or Skene's gland abscess

This is the result of obstruction of the affected gland ducts, causing pain, swelling and sometimes fever. Culture commonly yields a mixed growth. *N. gonorrhoeae* and *C. trachomatis* often cause bartholinitis, which should be borne in mind when assessing patients (see Chapter 2). Skin organisms such as *Staphylococcus* species may also be involved.

Epididymitis

Epididymitis is defined as inflammation of the epididymis triggered by an infectious agent (Table 7.3), and can extend to involve the testis (epididymo-orchitis). Symptoms and signs are commonly unilateral but may be bilateral.

Clinical findings include scrotal swelling, erythema and pain. Examination will usually reveal unilateral or bilateral testicular discomfort, with tender swollen epididymides.

Diagnosis is essentially clinical. There may be a history of urethral discharge and dysuria.

Differential diagnoses are usually unilateral presentations. The most important is torsion, which becomes less common after 20 years of age.

TABLE 7.3

Infectious agents that cause epididymitis

Agent	Comment
Neisseria gonorrhoeae	Up to 15% also have C. trachomatis
Chlamydia trachomatis	Most common cause under 35 years of age
Escherichia coli	Usually occurs in those over 35 years of age
Enterobacteriaceae	Patients may have structural urinary tract abnormality
Mycobacterium tuberculosis	Chronic epididymitis (rare in developed countries)
Fungal infection (histoplasmosis, blastomycosis, coccidiomycosis, cryptococcosis)	Chronic epididymitis (rare)

If there is any doubt, scrotal exploration should be considered because of the risk of irreversible damage after 4 hours of torsion. Other differential diagnoses include inguinal hernia and tumor. Although the latter is relatively rare, as the presenting age group is 20–30 years of age, clinicians should consider further evaluation if there is no response to therapy.

Assessment. The patient should be screened for STIs (see Table 2.4, page 17), and a urine dipstick test performed and a midstream urine sample cultured.

Management. In men under the age of 35 years, the cause is more likely to be an STI, and therapy should cover this possibility while microbiological results are awaited. Ofloxacin is the antibiotic of choice for all age groups in the primary care setting, and will cover STIs and non-STIs (Table 7.4). Treatment should be for at least 2 weeks. Rest, simple analgesics and supportive underwear may also help recovery.

TABLE 7.4

Treatment guidelines for epididymitis

Recommended regimens	Alternative regimens	Contact treatment
Infection likely to be gonococcal		
• Antigonococcal treatment plus doxycycline, 100 mg twice daily for 10–14 days	• Ofloxacin, 200 mg twice daily, or 400 mg once daily for 10–14 days • Levofloxacin, 250 mg* once daily for 10–14 days	• Manage as gonococcal contact (see Table 9.4, page 72)
Infection likely to be chlamydial or caused by other non-gonococcal, non-enteric organisms		
• Doxycycline, 100 mg twice daily for 10–14 days	• Ofloxacin, 200 mg twice daily, or 400 mg once daily for 10–14 days • Levofloxacin, 250 mg* once daily for 10–14 days	• Treat as non-specific genital infection (see Table 3.3, page 30)
Infection likely to be caused by enteric organisms		
• Ofloxacin, 200 mg twice daily, or 400 mg once daily for 10–14 days	• Levofloxacin, 250 mg* once daily for 10–14 days	

*500 mg in US guideline.

Contact tracing/partner notification. Current and recent partners (a minimum of 30–60 days) should be traced and treated unless a urinary pathogen is isolated.

Follow-up. The patient should be reviewed at 2 weeks; therapy can be continued for up to 1 month if he is not fully recovered. The patient should be advised that full recovery may take some time; symptoms may take longer to resolve than eradication of active infection. Epididymitis is a late manifestation of infection and may take several months or longer to develop. If the patient does not respond to therapy, re-examine to ensure there is no structural abnormality, and reassess to check:

- antibiotic compliance
- partner treatment
- avoidance of sexual intercourse
- risk of reinfection
- use of analgesics.

Key points – pelvic inflammatory disease and epididymo-orchitis

- Pelvic infection is a clinical diagnosis and is not dependent on a positive infection test.
- If pelvic inflammatory disease (PID) is suspected, treatment should be prescribed. Public health strategies intentionally overdiagnose because of infertility implications.
- The causative agent in pelvic infection and epididymo-orchitis in men under 35 years of age is most commonly a sexually transmitted pathogen; partner(s) must be screened and treated.
- The risk of infertility in women increases significantly with repeated infection. The most common reason for repeated infection is failure to treat a sexual partner.
- Treatment regimens for PID and epididymo-orchitis must include an effective antichlamydial antibiotic.

All branches of medicine have a group of patients with symptoms that may be characteristic of physical disease but that are not associated with evidence of pathology, including regional pain syndromes. In sexual medicine there is now a well-recognized group of disorders that fit into this category – the genital pain syndromes. In women these include the vulval pain syndromes or vulvodynia and some cases of chronic pelvic pain. In men these include chronic pelvic pain syndrome (CPPS), sometimes known as chronic prostatitis, and chronic testicular pain.

Both sexes may present with urethral and/or bladder symptoms. Where no infection is found, this group of conditions is referred to as interstitial cystitis and/or the urethral syndrome in women, and in men this is usually part of the spectrum of CPPS presentations, sometimes called chronic non-specific urethritis (NSU).

Differential diagnoses

Any evidence of another pathology that might explain the symptoms should be investigated and treated before making a diagnosis of a genital pain syndrome, although both diagnoses will sometimes coexist. The main differential diagnoses include infection (STI/non-sexually transmitted infection) and genital skin disease. A full history, careful examination and simple screening tests for infection should exclude a treatable underlying condition. Sometimes such screening tests will need to be repeated when the patient is most symptomatic to ensure that diagnoses such as recurrent candidiasis or recurrent urinary tract infections are not missed.

Diagnosis

Pain syndromes are diagnoses of exclusion and are often made late in patients who may have had many medical consultations over months or years. Where a patient has persistent symptoms despite apparently adequate treatment, or no evidence of other specific diagnoses, then the diagnosis of a pain syndrome may be appropriate.

The symptoms and signs (Table 8.1) reflect the site affected and are quite variable, commonly relapsing and remitting, and may have been present for months or years.

Management

Establishing the diagnosis is highly therapeutic for many patients. It is also important to stress that, for the majority of patients, symptoms resolve over time. Strategies for managing chronic pain with low doses of tricyclic drugs used for their analgesic effects, for example, may accelerate recovery. Where there are also sexual problems, a combined management approach with a psychosexual specialist may also help. Full guidance about management is beyond the scope of this text. Initial assessment and treatment may require referral to a specialist.

TABLE 8.1

Signs and symptoms of common genital pain syndromes

Common symptoms	Signs
Vulval pain syndromes	
• Vulval burning/itching • Entry dyspareunia • Pain after intercourse • Discomfort riding a bicycle	• Often none • Touch tenderness (cotton bud causes pain when the introitus is touched)
Male pelvic pain syndromes (including chronic prostatitis)	
• Pelvic pain • Penile tip pain • Pain at the root of the penis • Ejaculatory pain • Testicular pain	• Often none • Some discomfort at the root and tip of the penis when the prostate is massaged
Female interstitial cystitis/urethral syndrome	
• Frequency • Dysuria	• Often none • Abnormal urine dipstick test should be investigated

Key points – genital pain syndromes

- Genital pain syndromes are diagnoses of exclusion; any definite abnormalities should be fully investigated.
- For most patients symptoms improve with time, but expert assessment and initial management may improve outcome.
- Diagnosis is often delayed, partly because symptoms can relapse and remit. There may be a history of repeated consultations and treatments for conditions such as candidiasis, recurrent urinary tract infection or non-specific urethritis without good evidence of infection.

9 Bacterial infections

Sexually transmitted bacterial infections include:
- *Chlamydia*
- gonorrhea
- bacterial vaginosis (may not be sexually transmitted)
- syphilis
- chancroid
- lymphogranuloma venereum
- granuloma inguinale (donovanosis)
- genital mycoplasmas.

Chlamydia trachomatis (excluding lymphogranuloma venereum)

C. trachomatis is an obligate intracellular bacterium with a long lifecycle. Serotypes D to K are responsible for the common infections of the human genital tract.

Transmission is sexual in adults. The incubation period preceding symptomatic infection is usually 7–21 days; however, asymptomatic infection can persist for long periods, with symptoms developing either spontaneously or when an intervention (e.g. insertion of an intrauterine device) leads to complicated infection such as pelvic inflammatory disease (PID).

Clinical features. Women with uncomplicated infection are usually asymptomatic, but may complain of abnormal vaginal discharge (often caused by concomitant vaginal pathogens), menstrual irregularities, dysuria or pelvic pain. They may have mucopurulent cervicitis (Figure 9.1). The most common symptoms in men are dysuria and/or urethral discharge, but many – at least 50% – are asymptomatic. Rectal infection (uncommon in heterosexuals) is usually asymptomatic, as is pharyngeal infection.

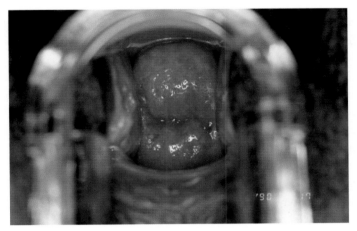

Figure 9.1 Chlamydial cervicitis with cervical friability, edema and ectopy.

The findings from physical examination are often normal in both men and women (Table 9.1).

TABLE 9.1
Signs of chlamydial infection

Men
- No signs (up to 50%)
- Meatitis
- Urethral discharge and/or dysuria (approximately 50%)
- Local complications, such as epididymitis (approximately 2%)

Women
- No signs (up to 70%)
- Cervicitis with evidence of cervical friability, mucopurulent discharge, contact bleeding (up to 50%)
- Local complications (up to 10%)
  - bartholinitis
  - skenitis
  - adnexal tenderness
  - cervical motion tenderness (cervical excitation)

Complications. In men, the most common complication of untreated infection is epididymitis (see Chapter 7). The potential consequences of ascending infection in women are shown in Table 9.2. A recent study from Sweden puts the risk of developing PID in women who had ever tested positive for *Chlamydia* at 5.6%. Up to one-third of upper genital tract disease is asymptomatic or subsymptomatic (i.e. non-specific). The risk of infertility increases with each episode of PID and may be as high as 60–75% after three episodes of PID. Perihepatitis (FitzHugh–Curtis syndrome) and reactive seronegative arthritis may occur. Autoinoculation may result in chlamydial conjunctivitis. As with most STIs, chlamydial infection can facilitate transmission of human immunodeficiency virus (HIV).

Diagnosis. *C. trachomatis* infection was traditionally diagnosed by cell culture, but this is expensive and time-consuming, and few laboratories still offer this service. Culture is the recommended method for detecting *C. trachomatis* at all exposed sites following sexual assault in adults because of 100% specificity, although the sensitivity is probably no more than 75%, even under ideal conditions. The use of nucleic acid amplification tests (NAATs) in forensics is evolving.

Currently, NAATs are the best available tests, with good sensitivity and specificity – they are the tests of choice for urethral, cervical and first-catch urine specimens (first 15–50 mL urine passed at any time of the day, as long as the patient has not urinated for at least 1 hour).

TABLE 9.2

Potential consequences of ascending chlamydial infection in women

- Endometritis with intermenstrual/postcoital bleeding
- Salpingitis/pelvic inflammatory disease
- Tubal damage
- Ectopic pregnancy
- Acute and chronic pelvic pain
- Infertility

However, sensitivity is affected by a number of factors, including inhibitors, contamination and oral contraceptive use.

Both male and female urethral samples and cervical samples are suitable for all tests. Most NAATs are licensed for use on first-catch urine for men and women, although these tests are less sensitive than those on urethral or endocervical specimens. Vulval–vaginal samples have been shown to produce equivalent sensitivity to endocervical testing for use with NAATs, and some kits are now licensed. NAATs for rectal samples are being evaluated; for centers without access to culture, this is the test of choice for rectal samples.

Treatment. An adequate dose of effective antibiotics should be given in a dosing regimen that will maximize compliance (Table 9.3). Single-dose regimens are preferred where feasible. Patients should not have sexual intercourse, even using condoms, until they have completed their treatment and their sexual partners have been treated. Other STIs should be sought and treated.

Pregnancy. Chlamydial infection is associated with low birth weight and postpartum endometritis, as well as neonatal conjunctivitis and pneumonitis. Perinatal transmission results in neonatal conjunctivitis in 30–50% of exposed babies, usually presenting in the second week of life. Less commonly, chlamydial infection causes pneumonitis, which presents between 4 and 12 weeks of age. Because the choice of antibiotic in pregnancy is limited, pregnant women should be followed carefully to exclude treatment failure and reinfection. Recent data suggest that chlamydial infection is more prevalent in women undergoing termination of pregnancy, and testing is recommended in this group. In some clinics, the rates are high enough to justify pre-emptive treatment in all women undergoing pregnancy termination.

Follow-up is important to:
- ensure that partner notification has taken place
- check compliance
- exclude reinfection.

TABLE 9.3

Treatment guidelines for uncomplicated chlamydial infection

Recommended regimens

- Doxycycline, 100 mg twice daily for 7 days (contraindicated in pregnancy)
- Azithromycin, 1 g orally in a single dose

Alternative regimens

(for use if the recommended treatments are contraindicated)

- Erythromycin, 500 mg twice daily for 10–14 days
- Ofloxacin,* 200 mg twice daily or 400 mg once daily for 7 days
- Levofloxacin, 500 mg once daily for 7 days[†]

Regimen in pregnancy

- Erythromycin, 500 mg four times daily for 7 days or twice daily for 14 days
- Amoxicillin, 500 mg three times daily for 7 days
- Azithromycin, 1 g as a single dose[‡]

Contact treatment

- Use recommended regimens

*Ofloxacin has similar efficacy to doxycycline and a better side-effect profile but is considerably more expensive, so is not recommended as first-line treatment. Dose recommended in US guideline is 300 mg.
[†]US guideline.
[‡]The safety of azithromycin during pregnancy and breastfeeding has not yet been fully assessed, although available data indicate that it is safe. World Health Organization guidelines recommend 1 g immediately to treat *Chlamydia trachomatis* in pregnancy; the *British National Formulary* recommends its use during pregnancy and breastfeeding only if no alternative is available.

Routine tests of cure are not indicated if standard treatment has been given, there is confirmation that the patient has adhered to therapy and there is no risk of reinfection, except in pregnant women, where a test of cure is desirable. If a test of cure is performed, it should be undertaken 3–5 weeks after completion of treatment. The non-culture tests can have false-positive results up to 3 weeks after treatment.

Contact tracing/partner notification. It is important that all sexual partners in at least the previous 3 months, or the previous partner if longer since partner change, are seen and treated, irrespective of their *Chlamydia* test result.

Gonorrhea

Neisseria gonorrhoeae is a Gram-negative diplococcus that infects mucosal surfaces of the genital tract, rectum, oropharynx and eye. It is a delicate organism that endures poorly out of the body, does not survive drying and is fastidious in its growth requirements.

Transmission. Gonorrhea is always sexually transmitted in adults. Transmission is more efficient from men to women than vice versa, and the risk of acquisition from a single act of sexual intercourse is estimated at 30–70%. Vertical transmission also occurs. An expert should investigate any incidence of gonorrhea in infants or children and involve the relevant authorities, because of the possibility of sexual abuse.

Clinical features. Symptoms and signs of gonorrhea depend on the site(s) of infection, which in turn depend on the sexual lifestyle of the patient. Men with urethral infection typically develop symptoms, most commonly discharge or discharge with dysuria, 2–10 days after exposure (Figure 9.2), although this takes longer in a proportion (up to 15%), and some remain asymptomatic. Although rectal infection can cause rectal/anal pain or discharge, it is usually asymptomatic. Rectal infection can occur in women in the absence of anal intercourse. Cervical infection is asymptomatic in about 70% of episodes, and the symptoms that do occur, such as vaginal discharge and low abdominal or pelvic pain, are non-specific for gonorrhea. Pharyngeal infection is usually asymptomatic, although pharyngitis may develop.

Examination may be normal, although signs may be observed depending on the site of infection. The most common finding in men is urethral discharge, which can vary from scant and mucoid to copious and purulent. The most commonly observed signs in women are

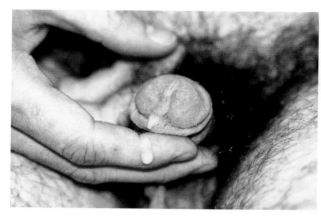

Figure 9.2
Gonococcal
urethral
discharge.

mucopurulent cervicitis and vaginal discharge. The discharge is
often the result of concomitant infection; gonococcal discharge has
no pathognomonic features. Signs of local complications may be
present in both sexes.

Complications occur more commonly when untreated infection
has been present for a prolonged period. Complications occur in
approximately 3% of women and fewer than 1% of men in the UK,
but higher rates are reported in the USA, with 5–20% of untreated
women developing gonococcal PID. Infection can facilitate HIV
transmission in both sexes.

    Local complications in men include:
- paraurethral duct infection
- tysonitis
- periurethral abscess
- penile edema and lymphangitis
- ascending local infection of the epididymides.

    Local complications in women include:
- bartholinitis/skenitis (Figure 9.3)
- endometritis
- salpingitis, which may lead to peritonitis and tubo-ovarian
  abscesses.

    Much less commonly, disseminated infection occurs in both sexes by
hematogenous spread. In such cases, complications may include:

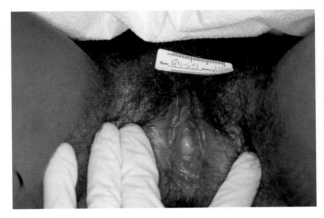

Figure 9.3
Skenitis
(Skene's gland
abscess),
similar to
bartholinitis.

- septicemia
- arthritis
- dermatitis
- endocarditis
- meningitis.

Skin lesions are most commonly seen on distal extremities and begin as papules or petechiae before evolving into microseptic pustular infarcts. There are seldom more than five or six lesions. Arthritis is typically polyarticular arthritis or tenosynovitis, most commonly involving the knees, wrists, small joints of the hands, ankles and elbows. Endocarditis and meningitis have become very rare and are most often seen in individuals with a deficiency in one of the components of the complement pathway.

Diagnosis. Immediate Gram-stained microscopy will detect up to 98% of symptomatic urethral infections in men, but only 50–70% of asymptomatic infections. Microscopy of specimens from the cervix and rectum is less reliable (40–50%), and microscopy of oropharyngeal specimens is unhelpful. NAATs are gradually replacing culture as the preferred diagnostic medium in many settings. Culture of the gonococcus, when performed, also provides information on antibiotic sensitivities. Specimens from all sites can be cultured for *N. gonorrhoeae*. Culture has been reported to have a sensitivity for urethral and endocervical infection of 85–95% and, with confirmation, has a specificity of 100% and positive predictive value (PPV) of 100%. NAAT specimens can also be first-void urine samples (i.e. first urine sample of the morning). The NAATs available have a sensitivity comparable to that of culture, estimated to be 92.1% and 96.4% for endocervical and urethral specimens, respectively, and the PPV is less than 100%.

In most women, the diagnosis is made by NAAT from a cervical smear, a self-administered vaginal swab or urine sample. Culture, when performed, is of a sample obtained from the endocervix, cultured on selective medium. In women who have had a hysterectomy, urethral culture offers a better yield than high vaginal culture. If a Bartholin's abscess is present, expressed material can be Gram-stained for microscopy and evaluated. In high-risk women (contacts of patients diagnosed with gonorrhea), additional samples should be taken from all possible sites of infection (oropharynx, urethra and rectum).

In men who have sex with men, rectal cultures should be obtained if there is a history of oro–anal or anogenital contact, ideally under direct vision of the rectal mucosa (i.e. using a proctoscope). The oropharynx should be sampled in all gonorrhea contacts and in homosexual men. NAATs have not been fully evaluated for rectal or pharyngeal sites.

A full set of genital tests is advised in patients with suspected disseminated infection. The diagnosis may be made on blood culture or culture of joint aspirate, but both lack sensitivity compared with genital sampling in patients with disseminated infection. It must be remembered that these patients have an STI. They should be advised accordingly, and their sexual contacts sought and investigated.

In cases of sexual assault or infection in children, culture is the recommended method for detecting N. gonorrhoeae because of 100% specificity.

Patients at high risk of gonorrhea who are not treated on an epidemiological basis (treatment given to named contacts of patients after a history of exposure to disease but without, or in advance of, confirmatory pathological findings) should have samples taken on two occasions before a diagnosis of gonorrhea can be excluded.

Treatment. The aims of treatment are to eliminate the organism from all sites and to minimize the risk of complications and the potential for transmission. Treatment for uncomplicated genital infection should eradicate more than 95% of infections. The choice of antibiotic should be guided by known local gonococcal sensitivities. Gonococcal antibiotic resistance has become an increasing problem in recent years; N. gonorrhoeae has evolved a number of resistance mechanisms, including beta-lactamase plasmid and chromosomally mediated penicillin resistance, plasmid and chromosomally mediated tetracycline resistance and chromosomally mediated quinolone resistance. Resistance to macrolides has also been demonstrated, and sporadic high-level chromosomally mediated spectinomycin resistance has been described. Patients who acquired the infection in south-east Asia are at greatest risk for multidrug-resistant infection.

To improve compliance, a single supervised dose of antibiotic should be given where possible (Table 9.4). Sexual abstinence should be advised until sexual partners have been treated. Disseminated infection should be treated with the same antibiotics as used in uncomplicated infections. Intra-articular instillation of antibiotics is unnecessary in the treatment of gonococcal arthritis.

Coexisting infections should be sought and treated appropriately. Chlamydial coinfection is common in both men and women with gonorrhea; concurrent treatment is therefore recommended.

Pregnancy. Approximately 30% of babies who are born to infected mothers but do not receive prophylaxis develop gonococcal ophthalmia neonatorum.

Neonatal sepsis may occur, particularly when there has been prolonged rupture of membranes or preterm delivery. Pregnant women should not be treated with quinolone or tetracycline antimicrobials.

Follow-up. Patients should be assessed after treatment. A test of cure is not routinely necessary when infection has been treated with a recommended directly observed therapy, symptoms have resolved and there is no risk of reinfection. A test of cure with culture should take

71

TABLE 9.4

Treatment guidelines for uncomplicated anogenital gonococcal infection

Recommended regimens*

- Ceftriaxone, 250 mg intramuscularly as a single dose
- Cefixime, 400 mg orally as a single dose
- Spectinomycin, 2 g intramuscularly as a single dose[†]

Alternative regimens

(when antimicrobial sensitivity is known or where regional prevalence of resistance to these antimicrobials is known to be <5%)

- Ciprofloxacin, 500 mg orally as a single dose[‡]
- Ofloxacin, 400 mg orally as a single dose[‡]
- Ampicillin, 2 or 3 g, plus probenecid 1 g orally as a single dose

Regimen in pregnancy

- Ceftriaxone, 250 mg intramuscularly as a single dose
- Cefixime, 400 mg orally as a single dose
- Spectinomycin, 2 g intramuscularly as a single dose[†]
- Ampicillin, 2 or 3 g, plus probenecid, 1 g orally as a single dose (where regional prevalence of resistance to these antimicrobials is known to be <5%)
- Pregnant women should not be treated with quinolone or tetracycline antimicrobials

Contact treatment

- Use recommended regimen if treating on epidemiological grounds

*In some areas of the world, such as the Far East and Pacific Islands, there are high rates of resistance to quinolones and penicillin. The US Centers for Disease Control recommend that patients with gonorrhea acquired in these areas should not be treated with quinolone-based regimens.
[†]Spectinomycin is not available in the USA.
[‡]Recommended regimen in the US guideline.

place 48–72 hours after the last antibiotic has been administered if the patient is symptomatic or received a suboptimal treatment, a potentially resistant strain is identified on culture or there is a possibility of reinfection.

Contact tracing/partner notification. It is essential that all recent (in at least the past 3 months) and current sexual partners are seen and tested for gonorrhea. In some situations, epidemiological treatment may be given; this is justified if the risk of unnecessary treatment is outweighed by the risk of complications of the infection or the likelihood of infecting others. The mother of a neonate diagnosed with gonococcal ophthalmitis, and her sexual partners, must be seen and managed as gonococcal contacts.

Bacterial vaginosis

Bacterial vaginosis is a common condition characterized by an overgrowth of predominantly anaerobic organisms (e.g. *Gardnerella vaginalis*, *Orevotella* spp., *Mycoplasma hominis*, *Mobiluncus* spp.) in the vagina, leading to a replacement of lactobacilli and an increase in vaginal pH.

Transmission. There is increasing debate about sexual transmission of bacterial vaginosis. Bacterial vaginosis can arise and remit spontaneously in women regardless of sexual activity, although it is seen almost exclusively in women who have been sexually active.

Clinical features. Approximately 50% of women are asymptomatic, but bacterial vaginosis may cause an offensive, fishy-smelling vaginal discharge. Occasionally mild low abdominal pain can occur. Examination may reveal a thin, white, homogeneous discharge.

Complications. There is an association with PID, preterm delivery, low birth-weight babies and post-termination endometritis. Recent studies suggest that bacterial vaginosis may facilitate HIV transmission.

Diagnosis

Amsel's criteria (Table 9.5) are simple to perform, and require minimal materials other than a microscope. However, the disadvantages are that the patient must undergo a vaginal examination, and the

TABLE 9.5

Amsel's criteria for the diagnosis of bacterial vaginosis

The presence of three of the following is sufficient for a diagnosis:

- thin, white homogeneous discharge at vaginal examination
- clue cells on microscopy
- vaginal fluid pH > 4.5
- positive whiff test (release of fishy odor on adding 10% potassium hydroxide)

recognition of the vaginal discharge and the fishy smell has a subjective endpoint.

The whiff test is still performed in US clinics but is falling out of favor in the UK because of the caustic nature of potassium hydroxide. Without the whiff test, the method is invalidated, as it depends on measurement of all four Amsel's criteria to achieve a high sensitivity.

A Gram-stained vaginal smear is an alternative means of diagnosis. The relative proportions of bacteriological morphotypes are estimated – a paucity of lactobacilli (Gram-positive bacilli) and a preponderance of Gram-negative bacilli and coccobacillary organisms indicate bacterial vaginosis. It has the advantage of a more objective endpoint, although a microscope is required. A number of simplified schemes have been described: the Ison–Hay method (Table 9.6) of grading vaginal flora gives a good correlation with Amsel's criteria for the diagnosis of bacterial vaginosis and correlates well with other scoring methods.

Treatment (Table 9.7) is recommended for symptomatic women, those undergoing certain surgical procedures and pregnant women. Treatment of asymptomatic women is more controversial.

Pregnancy. Bacterial vaginosis is associated with late miscarriage, preterm birth, premature (preterm) rupture of membranes and postpartum endometritis.

TABLE 9.6

Appearance of Gram-stained smear according to the modified Ison–Hay scoring system for the diagnosis of bacterial vaginosis

Grade 0   Epithelial cells with no bacteria

Grade I   Normal vaginal flora (*Lactobacillus* morphotypes alone)

Grade II   Reduced numbers of *Lactobacillus* morphotypes with a mixed bacterial flora

Grade III   Mixed bacterial flora only, few or absent *Lactobacillus* morphotypes

Grade IV   Gram-positive cocci only

Grade III is consistent with bacterial vaginosis as diagnosed by Amsel's criteria (Table 9.5); thus, only grade III flora indicates bacterial vaginosis.

TABLE 9.7

Treatment guidelines for bacterial vaginosis

Recommended regimens

- Metronidazole, 400–500 mg twice daily for 5–7 days
- Metronidazole, 2 g in a single dose*

Alternative regimens

- Metronidazole 0.75% gel, intravaginally once daily for 5 days
- Clindamycin 2% cream, intravaginally once daily for 7 days, or clindamycin 100 g ovules, intravaginally at bedtime for 3 days
- Clindamycin, 300 mg twice daily for 7 days
- Tinidazole, 2 g as a single dose

Regimen in pregnancy

- Metronidazole, 400–500 mg twice daily for 5–7 days
- Metronidazole 0.75% gel, intravaginally once daily for 5 days*
- Clindamycin 2% cream, intravaginally once daily for 7 days
- Clindamycin, 300 mg twice daily for 7 days

*Not recommended in the US guideline.

Follow-up is not required if symptoms resolve, but recurrence is common (up to 50% by 3 months).

Contact tracing/partner notification is not required.

Syphilis

Syphilis is a multistage disease caused by the bacterium *Treponema pallidum*, a spirochete with a number of microbiological characteristics that influence its epidemiology and clinical management.

Transmission is almost exclusively sexual, although bacteria can be transmitted via blood transfusions and from mother to baby during pregnancy and breastfeeding. Sexual transmission occurs in the first 2 years of untreated infection, though transmission to a fetus may occur up to 10 years after the primary infection. Initial infection occurs through sexual contact at a mucosal membrane. The risk of acquisition from a contact with early syphilis is estimated to be 30%.

Clinical features. After the initial exposure, there is a latency period of 9–90 days before symptoms develop. The primary lesion is a macule, which becomes papular and then ulcerates to form the primary chancre (Table 9.8 and Figure 9.4). The ulcer is characteristically single, painless and indurated in the anogenital region, and may be accompanied by regional lymphadenopathy. Up to 50% are atypical in some way (e.g. multiple, painful, purulent or extragenital). Left untreated, the chancre will heal spontaneously in 2–6 weeks.

Syphilis is a systemic disease and dissemination can occur at any stage. In some studies, 10–15% of patients with early primary syphilis have cerebrospinal fluid abnormalities. The secondary syphilis syndrome develops 4–8 weeks after the primary lesion (see Table 9.8). The clinical features of secondary syphilis result from a systemic vasculitis caused by high levels of *T. pallidum* in the blood and associated immunologic responses. The manifestations of secondary syphilis include:
- rash
- alopecia

TABLE 9.8

Stages of syphilis

Stage	Incubation period	Signs
Primary	9–90 days	Painless ulcer
Secondary	2–6 months	Transient variable skin rash that can affect soles and palms (75%) Generalized lymphadenopathy (50%) Condylomata lata (warty-type lesions) on the genitals Mucosal ulceration of the mouth, throat, genitals (30%) Visceral syndromes (<10%)
Latent		Serological diagnosis (no clinical features)
Late	2–50 years after primary infection	Cardiovascular syphilis Neurosyphilis Late benign syphilis (gumma)

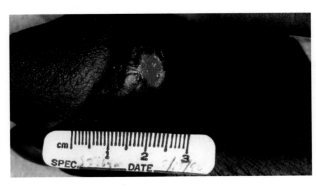

Figure 9.4
Primary
syphilis
chancre.

- generalized lymphadenopathy
- mucosal ulcers.

Of these, the most important is a generalized polymorphic rash, which characteristically involves the palms and soles. In contrast to the rash caused by rheumatologic disorders, the rash associated with secondary syphilis crosses the palmar creases.

77

Although not a common occurrence, the internal organs may become involved, and the following can occur:
- granulomatous hepatitis
- nephrotic syndrome
- optic neuritis
- meningovascular syphilis.

Left untreated, the secondary syphilis syndrome resolves spontaneously, usually within 1–2 months of onset. In the majority of infected patients, the symptoms and signs of early syphilis will pass unnoticed, or be so minor that a medical opinion is not sought.

Complications. Most patients not diagnosed or treated in the secondary stage will progress to latent syphilis. Early latent syphilis is a serological diagnosis defined by a fourfold increase in titer occurring within 2 years in the UK (1 year in the USA) of infection with no clinical evidence of disease. Late latent syphilis is a serological diagnosis of syphilis occurring more than 2 years (1 year in the USA) after infection. The late complications of syphilis, such as neurosyphilis, cardiovascular syphilis and gummatous syphilis, do not usually develop until 10–20 years (range 2–50 years) after acquisition of the infection, and are now very rare in most countries.

There is an epidemiological association between HIV infection and syphilis. All stages of syphilis are seen more commonly in HIV-positive patients, and studies in STI clinics have demonstrated that in these settings the prevalence of HIV infection is up to three times higher in patients with syphilis than in those without syphilis. Case reports suggest that late complications occur earlier in patients infected with HIV.

Diagnosis. *T. pallidum* cannot be grown in culture, and therefore the diagnosis of syphilis is based on clinical findings, microscopy and serology. In early disease, the diagnosis may be made by finding spirochetes in the exudate from lesions, using dark ground microscopy (DGM). Serological tests cannot differentiate syphilis from other treponemal infections (e.g. yaws).

Lesions. DGM of lesion exudate or lymph nodes performed by experienced clinicians can make the diagnosis in primary and secondary syphilis. DGM is not suitable for examining oral lesions and is less reliable for examining rectal and non-penile genital lesions.

The polymerase chain reaction (PCR) is useful in the diagnosis of primary syphilis and can be used on samples from sites where contamination with commensal treponemes is likely. It should soon become routinely available.

Serological screening tests. The serological diagnosis of syphilis is a two-step procedure. Initially, either a *T. pallidum* enzyme immunoassay or a non-treponemal screening test, such as the venereal disease research laboratory (VDRL) or rapid plasma reagin (RPR) test, is used. Results are reported as titers – the dilutions required to achieve a negative reaction using standard reagents. Patients with a positive non-treponemal test should have a confirmatory test, such as the fluorescent treponemal antibody-absorbed (FTA-ABS) or microhemagglutination (MHATP or HATS) tests. Up to 20% of patients with a positive screening test will have a negative confirmatory test. These are 'biological false positives' (Table 9.9). Biological false positives with titers above 1:16 are extremely unusual. Treponemal tests should not be used for routine screening.

In primary syphilis, the sensitivity of serological testing is 85%. False negatives occur because seroconversion may not take place until up to 2 weeks after the appearance of the primary lesion. In secondary syphilis, sensitivity of serological diagnosis is close to 100%, and titers may be extremely high. A false-negative test result may occur as a result of the prozone phenomenon from using undiluted serum, which occurs

TABLE 9.9

Causes of biological false positives in confirmatory tests for syphilis

- Pregnancy
- Connective tissue disorders
- Intravenous drug use
- Acute infectious process
- Chronic infectious process

in patients with very high RPR/VDRL titers, such that all the reagent sites become occupied. A positive test can be distinguished by diluting the serum.

The diagnosis of late syphilis is based on a combination of positive treponemal tests, with or without positive non-treponemal tests, and a careful clinical assessment. This should include a history focusing on previous treatment for syphilis, symptoms of early and late syphilis and a clinical examination.

Treatment. Parenteral penicillin is the first-line treatment for all stages of syphilis (Table 9.10). Treatment regimens are similar for most patients infected with HIV. Patients with positive syphilis serology but no history of adequate treatment should be treated as for active syphilis. Coexisting STIs should be sought and treated.

The Jarisch–Herxheimer reaction to treatment is a self-limiting, acute febrile illness that is common in early syphilis. It is not important except in pregnancy, when it may cause fetal distress and premature labor. Although uncommon in late syphilis, it is potentially life-threatening at this stage.

Procaine penicillin toxicity is uncommon and may present as either anxiety and hallucinations or, occasionally, circulatory collapse and convulsions. It results from inadvertent intra-arterial injection of procaine penicillin (used to treat syphilis in the UK but not in the USA). Symptoms are usually mild and will settle with reassurance. A few patients will need resuscitation, and appropriate facilities should be available when treatment with procaine penicillin is initiated.

Pregnancy. The vertical transmission rate in women who have untreated primary or secondary syphilis is 75–95%. In-utero infection may manifest either as stillbirth or as the stigmata of congenital syphilis, which include clinical syndromes at birth and osteoformative abnormalities, including 'sabre shins', Hutchinson's incisors and Moon's (mulberry) molars. Late congenital syphilis is rarely seen these days.

Follow-up. Individuals with early syphilis should be evaluated clinically and serologically at 3-monthly intervals for at least 1 year, to assess the effectiveness of treatment and to detect relapse or reinfection. Patients with late disease should be followed up annually for at least 3 years.

Contact tracing/partner notification. For patients with primary syphilis, sexual partners in the 3 months before diagnosis should be seen. Partner notification may have to extend to 6 months for patients with secondary syphilis and to 1–2 years for early latent syphilis. Serological tests for syphilis should be performed at the first visit and repeated at 6 weeks and 3 months. Individuals with late latent syphilis and late syphilis are generally not infectious to their sexual partners, although vertical transmission may occur up to 10 years after the initial infection. Current sexual partners should undergo serological screening with treponemal and non-treponemal tests, as should children born to women diagnosed with late latent or late syphilis of unknown duration.

Chancroid

Chancroid is caused by a Gram-negative coccobacillus, *Haemophilus ducreyi*. The disease is generally seen in tropical areas, including Africa, Asia, Latin America and the Caribbean, and is endemic in a few areas of the USA. It is rare in the UK, and infection is almost always acquired overseas. *H. ducreyi* infection should be considered in a patient with genital ulceration where there is a history of recent travel by the patient or their sexual partner to a part of the world where chancroid is endemic.

Transmission is sexual, though autoinoculation of extragenital sites has been described.

Clinical features. Chancroid is seen more commonly in men than in women. After a short incubation period of 2–8 days a papule develops that progresses to ulceration of the prepuce, frenum or glans penis (Figure 9.5, page 84). These are characteristically painful, soft, destructive lesions (unlike the indurated chancre of primary syphilis) with undermined ragged edges; the inguinal nodes are enlarged.

Complications. Advanced untreated infections may become secondarily infected, resulting in extensive destructive ulceration

TABLE 9.10

Treatment guidelines for syphilis

Recommended regimens	Alternative regimens

Primary, secondary and early latent syphilis

Recommended regimens	Alternative regimens
• Benzathine penicillin, 2.4 MU intramuscularly as a single dose (USA) or two doses at weekly intervals (UK) • Procaine penicillin G, 0.6 MU intramuscularly once daily for 10–14 days	• Doxycycline, 200 mg daily (either 100 mg twice daily or 200 mg as a single dose) for 14 days • Tetracycline, 500 mg four times daily for 14 days • Azithromycin, 500 mg daily for 10 days • Amoxicillin, 500 mg four times daily, plus probenecid, 500 mg four times daily for 14 days

Late latent syphilis/cardiovascular syphilis/gummata (assuming exclusion of asymptomatic neurosyphilis by cerebrospinal fluid examination)

Recommended regimens	Alternative regimens
• Benzathine penicillin, 2.4 MU intramuscularly as three doses at weekly intervals • Procaine penicillin G, 0.75 MU intramuscularly once daily for 17 days	• Doxycycline, 200 mg daily (either 100 mg twice daily or 200 mg as a single dose) for 30 days • Amoxicillin, 2 g orally three times daily, plus probenecid, 500 mg four times daily for 28 days

Neurosyphilis

Recommended regimens	Alternative regimens
• Procaine penicillin, 2 g intramuscularly once daily, plus probenecid, 500 mg orally four times daily for 17 days • Benzylpenicillin, 18–24 MU daily, given as 3–4 MU intravenously every 4 hours for 17 days	• Doxycycline, 200 mg daily (either 100 mg twice daily or 200 mg as a single dose) for 30 days • Amoxicillin, 2 g orally three times daily, plus probenecid, 500 mg four times daily for 28 days

Bacterial infections

Regimen in pregnancy	Contact treatment
• Procaine penicillin G, 0.6 MU intramuscularly once daily for 10–14 days • Erythromycin, 500 mg four times daily for 14 days • Azithromycin 500 mg daily for 10 days	If treating epidemiologically: • Benzathine penicillin, 2.4 MU intramuscularly as a single dose • Doxycycline, 200 mg daily (either 100 mg twice daily or 200 mg as a single dose) for 14 days
• Procaine penicillin G, 0.6 MU intramuscularly once daily for 14 days • Erythromycin, 500 mg four times daily for 14 days • Azithromycin, 500 mg once daily for 10 days	Treat only if found to have syphilis after evaluation
• Procaine penicillin G, 0.6 MU intramuscularly once daily for 14 days • Erythromycin, 500 mg four times daily for 14 days • Azithromycin, 500 mg daily for 10 days	Treat only if found to have syphilis after evaluation

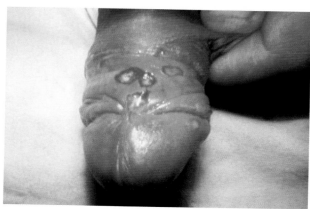

Figure 9.5 Chancroid with multiple ulcers. Differential diagnosis includes herpes simplex virus infection.

of the genital region, including development of buboes (Figure 9.6), with sinus formation. The presence of chancroid enhances HIV transmission.

Diagnosis. Because of the infrequency of requests, the laboratory diagnosis for chancroid is often unavailable and the diagnosis is often provisional, made if there is a response to a therapy trial. Ideally, the diagnosis is based on isolation of *H. ducreyi* from an ulcer or from pus aspirated from inguinal buboes, and the exclusion of other diseases with similar clinical manifestations. A culture result takes a minimum of 2 days and may take as long as 7 days to obtain (sensitivity varies from 33% in low-prevalence populations to 80% in high-prevalence populations). A Gram stain from the ulcer base has a low sensitivity and is not recommended as a diagnostic test.

There are no commercial NAATs available at present but molecular detection for *H. ducreyi* should be available in the future.

Treatment. Fluctuant nodes may need aspiration (Figure 9.6), or careful incision and drainage to prevent rupture and sinus tract formation. Effective antimicrobial therapy usually results in healing of the ulcer and resolution of the lymphadenopathy within 2 weeks (Table 9.11). High levels of resistance to treatment have been seen in HIV-infected individuals, who require longer courses. Other STIs should be sought and treated appropriately.

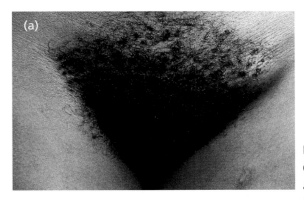

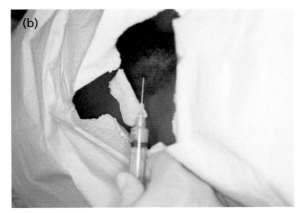

Figure 9.6
(a) Inguinal bubo
and
(b) aspiration of
chancroid/
lymphogranuloma
venereum bubo.

Pregnancy. No adverse effects of chancroid on pregnancy outcome or on the fetus have been reported. Vertical transmission is not described.

Follow-up. Relapse after treatment occurs in approximately 5% of patients; they will usually respond to a further course of the same antibiotics.

Contact tracing/partner notification. Sexual partners of the 10 days before the onset of symptoms should be screened and treated.

Lymphogranuloma venereum
The distinct *C. trachomatis* serovariants L1–L3 are responsible for lymphogranuloma venereum (LGV). Historically, most cases were

TABLE 9.11

Treatment guidelines for chancroid

Recommended regimens

- Azithromycin, 1 g as a single dose
- Ceftriaxone, 250 mg intramuscularly as a single dose
- Ciprofloxacin, 500 mg twice daily for 3 days
- Erythromycin, 500 mg four times daily for 7 days

Regimen in pregnancy

- Erythromycin, 500 mg four times daily for 7 days
- Ceftriaxone, 250 mg intramuscularly as a single dose

Contact treatment

- Use recommended regimens

diagnosed in those who had traveled to tropical and subtropical regions: Asia, Africa, South America or the Caribbean. Following outbreaks among men having sex with men in western Europe in 2003 and in some major US cities, however, LGV infections acquired in the UK and USA have been identified, and acquisition from abroad is more unusual.

Transmission. LGV is sexually transmitted, probably through minute abrasions or lacerations in the genital skin.

Clinical features. The primary lesion is a painless genital or rectal ulcer, which heals spontaneously in a few days. It is seen in 20–50% of infected men, but is rare in women. The lesion occurs early in the course of the disease (at 3–12 days), and is often unnoticed by the patient. Lymphangitis of the penis may develop. If rectal transmission occurs, the first manifestation may be an acute proctitis, with constipation, tenesmus and rectal discharge. Lymphadenopathy is rare but has been one of the presenting symptoms of recent cases in the UK.

Classically, most patients present at the second stage, which occurs between 10 days and 6 months after the initial infection, when the regional lymph nodes involved become firm, swollen and painful (i.e. buboes), although this has been uncommon in UK-acquired infections. Pelvic and retroperitoneal lymphadenopathy can occur in women and men with rectal LGV. The primary ulcerative lesions often resolve before or during this stage but proctitis is likely to persist. Constitutional disturbances, such as fever and malaise, commonly accompany local symptoms.

Complications arise following long-term untreated infection in up to 70% of individuals, and include fibrosis and abnormal lymphatic drainage. Depending on the site of infection, rectal strictures, anal fistulas or genital elephantiasis may occur. LGV is a cause of frozen pelvis and infertility.

Diagnosis. Routinely available NAATs for *C. trachomatis* will detect all serovars, including LGV serovars, and are licensed for genital specimens. In most patients now identified, rectal specimens need to be tested, and although there are no NAATs licensed for these samples, the available data support the validity of NAATs for use with rectal specimens. The presence of LGV-specific DNA can then be detected directly using real-time PCR. Culture is the most specific test but very few laboratories have culture facilities, and sensitivity may be lower for bubo aspirates.

Serology may be useful if direct detection has been unsuccessful. A high titer in a patient with symptoms is highly suggestive of LGV. However, a low titer cannot exclude LGV, and a high titer in the absence of symptoms cannot confirm LGV. The two methods most used have been complement fixation and microimmunofluorescence-immunoglobulin G; single-point titers of at least 1/64 and 1/256, respectively, are considered positive. Individuals with known or strongly suspected exposure to LGV can be retested 4 weeks after exposure if the initial test has been done within 3 weeks of exposure and epidemiological treatment has been declined.

Treatment. Fluctuant nodes should be aspirated through normal skin. In acute inflammation, incision and drainage or excision are contraindicated, as these techniques may cause complications such as fistula formation. The acute stage usually responds to appropriate oral antibiotics, although a prolonged course of treatment may be necessary (see Table 9.12). Without treatment, approximately 5% of individuals will develop the late sequelae of strictures and fistulas, which may require surgery. Other STIs should be sought and treated.

Pregnancy. There is no described adverse effect of LGV on pregnancy. Perinatal transmission has been documented.

Follow-up is important to monitor the response to treatment and to ensure that partners have been seen. Surgical intervention may be required for the very few patients who have extensive lesions or fistulas as a result of late treatment.

Contact tracing/partner notification. All sexual partners in the month preceding and during the symptomatic period should be examined and treated.

TABLE 9.12

Treatment guidelines for lymphogranuloma venereum

Recommended regimen
- Doxycycline, 100 mg twice daily for 21 days

Alternative regimen
- Erythromycin, 500 mg four times daily for 21 days

Regimen in pregnancy
- Erythromycin, 500 mg four times daily for 21 days

Contact treatment
- Use recommended regimen

Granuloma inguinale (donovanosis)

The causative organism is *Klebsiella granulomatis* (formerly known as *Donovania granulomatis* and *Calymmatobacterium granulomatis*), which occurs almost exclusively in tropical and subtropical regions. The disease is rarely reported in the UK and usually occurs in people who have lived in one of the endemic areas in India, Papua New Guinea, Brazil and South Africa or among Australian aboriginals.

Transmission is believed to be sexual, but the bacteria are not highly infectious. Transmission to infants during birth has been reported.

Clinical features. The incubation period is 9–90 days, after which the primary lesion develops. This firm papule or nodule develops into a painless indurated granulomatous ulcer, which is usually genital but may be oral, anal or at other extragenital locations. Prominent local lymphadenopathy usually ensues, often leading to further ulcerative lesions in the skin overlying the nodes involved.

Complications. Untreated, the primary infection may either resolve or spread locally to involve the whole of the external genitals, the inguinal area and the anus. Rarely, metastatic lesions occur on the back and breasts and in the liver and spleen. Healing leads to intense scarring and may result in genital lymphedema or genital mutilation. Malignant transformation can occur in longstanding lesions.

Diagnosis. A Leishman–Giemsa smear from the lesion will detect Donovan bodies in up to 95% of cases. Alternatively, the organisms may be detected on a biopsy specimen stained with a silver stain (e.g. Warthin–Starry) or Giemsa. Biopsy may be considered for smear-negative lesions, large lesions with easily removed friable tissue, any lesion where malignancy is suspected, and less common lesions of the mouth, anus, cervix and uterus.

Treatment. Until recently, protracted courses of antibiotics were advised, to be continued until the lesion had completely healed. However, recent data suggest that azithromycin for 1 week is sufficient to cure even extensive lesions. Current recommendations are for a minimum of 3 weeks' treatment (Table 9.13).

Investigation for other STIs should be performed.

Pregnancy. Children born to mothers with untreated genital lesions are at risk of infection. A course of prophylactic antibiotics should therefore be considered.

TABLE 9.13

Treatment guidelines for granuloma inguinale (donovanosis)*

Recommended regimens

- Azithromycin, 1 g weekly, or 500 mg daily
- Doxycyline, 100 mg twice daily
- Erythromycin, 500 mg four times daily
- Norfloxacin, 400 mg twice daily
- Co-trimoxazole, 160/800 mg combination twice daily
- Ceftriaxone, 1 g daily by intramuscular or intravenous injection

Alternative regimens

- Gentamicin sulfate, 1 mg/kg every 8 hours by intramuscular or intravenous injection as an adjunct to therapy in patients whose lesions do not respond in the first few days of treatment with other agents

Regimen in pregnancy

- Erythromycin, 500 mg four times daily
- Azithromycin, 1 g weekly or 500 mg daily
- Ceftriaxone, 1 g daily by intramuscular or intravenous injection

Contact treatment

- Use recommended regimen

*Treatment should be continued for a minimum of 3 weeks or until lesions have healed; healing times vary greatly between patients.

Follow-up. The patient should be followed up to ensure complete healing of lesions.

Contact tracing/partner notification. All sexual partners during the time of symptoms and in the 6 weeks before the development of symptoms should be examined and treated.

Genital mycoplasmas

Mycoplasma genitalium is probably an important pathogen in some men with non-gonococcal urethritis but commercial test kits are not currently available for its detection. The typical treatment strategies for non-gonococcal urethritis are effective against these organisms (see Table 3.3, page 30).

Key points – bacterial infections

- Bacterial STIs are frequently asymptomatic.
- Local and systemic complications may occur in untreated infections.
- STIs frequently coexist, so when one is diagnosed others should be sought and treated.
- An adequate dose of effective antibiotics should be given in a dosing regimen that will maximize compliance.
- Patients should not have sexual intercourse, even with condoms, until they have completed their treatment and their sexual partners have been treated.

Herpes simplex virus

There are two types of herpes simplex virus (HSV), HSV 1 and 2. HSV 2 is almost entirely associated with genital disease whereas HSV 1 is associated with both oropharyngeal and genital disease. Genital HSV 1 infection rates have been increasing. Recent studies in the UK suggest that in some areas HSV 1 accounts for over 50% of first episodes of genital herpes, as well as a large proportion of vertically transmitted neonatal herpes. Patients infected with HSV 1 have fewer symptomatic recurrences and less frequent subclinical shedding than those with HSV 2 infection.

Transmission. Herpes can only be transmitted when an infected individual is shedding virus, which can occur asymptomatically and when lesions are present (Figure 10.1). HSV is transmitted by close physical contact – sexual and/or orogenital – and occasionally by autoinoculation, for example to the eye. Infection is acquired through intact mucous membranes or when virus comes into contact with damaged keratinized epithelium.

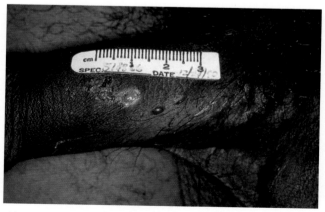

Figure 10.1 Herpes simplex virus lesions in various stages of development.

Clinical features. The clinical presentation is variable. A minority (probably fewer than 25%) will develop a severe primary attack (usually within 2–4 weeks of virus acquisition) or first clinical episode. It may not be possible to distinguish between a so-called primary attack (Figure 10.2), which implies a first infection with herpesvirus, and a first clinical episode, in which the patient may have acquired genital herpes at some time in the past but has only recently developed symptoms. Some patients develop only minor lesions, while 70–80% of individuals have no clinical symptoms and are diagnosed only when a sexual partner presents with symptoms. Infected persons shed the virus intermittently, regardless of whether lesions are clinically apparent.

Primary infection is usually more severe in women. The following symptoms may be present in both sexes:

- febrile illness (prodrome), lasting 5–7 days
- dysuria, urinary frequency
- painful inguinal lymphadenopathy
- tingling/neuropathic pain
- genital blisters, ulcers and/or fissures (Figure 10.3)
- headache.

An untreated first episode may last 3 weeks or longer.

Clinical course. The risk of symptomatic recurrence after a primary or first episode is increased in young patients (under 20 years of age), those who have a severe first episode and those with genital HSV-2

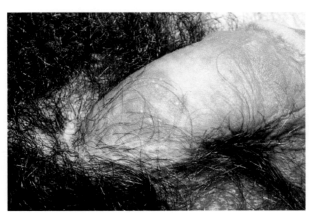

Figure 10.2
Intact herpes simplex virus vesicles.

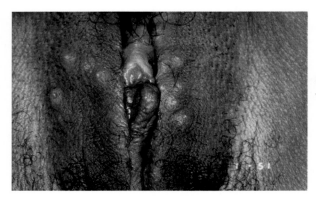

Figure 10.3
Vulvar herpes.

infection. The risk of recurrence is also higher in the first 3 months after a primary attack. Patients with HIV infection and evidence of immune deterioration (such as a declining CD4 count, rising viral load, or an acquired immune deficiency syndrome (AIDS)-defining illness) may develop more frequent and/or more severe recurrences.

Recurrent episodes are often mild and infrequent. Presenting symptoms in men and women typically include:

- neuropathic prodrome with, for example, tingling and/or burning, usually affecting the same region
- erythema, blisters, fissures and ulcers.

These usually resolve fully within 3–4 days.

Complications usually only arise with the first episode. The risk is reduced with early diagnosis and immediate systemic antiviral therapy. Complications can include:

- acute urinary retention (predominantly in women)
- constipation, which may be a risk with first-episode perianal disease
- aseptic meningitis.

Genital herpes is a life-long infection that can cause substantial morbidity to infected individuals and can have serious consequences, including neonatal herpes and increased risk for HIV acquisition and transmission.

Diagnosis. Patients should be seen as soon as possible during an acute episode to confirm the diagnosis. Swabs should be taken directly from lesions for either polymerase chain reaction (PCR) testing or culture of HSV, depending on local arrangements. PCR has HSV detection rates 11–71% higher than those of virus culture and may allow less stringent conditions for sample storage and transport. First-episode ulcers more often yield the virus than recurrent lesions (82% versus 43%).

Negative tests do not exclude the diagnosis in patients with a highly suggestive clinical history. Repeat testing with a future episode is indicated, and serological screening should be considered in patients with a history of recurrent genital symptoms of unknown etiology when direct virus detection methods (e.g. virus culture or PCR testing of genital specimens) have repeatedly yielded negative results. The diagnosis in patients with no history of clinical symptoms is difficult. Up to 50% of apparently asymptomatic patients will recall one or more episodes of genital symptoms suggestive of herpes. These patients should be encouraged to attend immediately they have symptoms in order to have herpes tests from the lesion(s).

Type-specific serum antibody testing for HSV 1 and 2 is available, and may help in the management of presumed asymptomatic carriers (frequently the contacts of index cases with primary herpes), in a patient with recurrent ulceration and repeatedly negative tests for herpes from the ulcer, and when advising discordant couples in pregnancy. HSV-2 antibodies are indicative of genital herpes whereas HSV-1 antibodies do not differentiate between genital and oropharyngeal infection. If an asymptomatic pregnant woman has a partner with a history of genital herpes, it may be useful to know her antibody status to advise about sexual contact during the pregnancy. If she does not have antibodies, sexual abstinence will prevent primary infection in pregnancy.

Treatment for genital herpes (Table 10.1) provides symptomatic relief but is not curative. Prompt treatment accelerates the time to healing, viral shedding and duration of symptoms. It does not, however, influence the likelihood of recurrences.

Primary/first episode. Start oral therapy immediately if the patient presents within 5 days of lesions developing, or after 5 days but with new lesions still forming.

TABLE 10.1

Treatment guidelines for genital herpes

Recommended regimens	Regimen in pregnancy	Contact treatment
Acute therapy (usually only indicated for primary infection/first episode)		
• Aciclovir, 200 mg five times daily for 5 days • Valaciclovir, 500 mg twice daily for 5 days • Famciclovir, 125 mg twice daily for 5 days	• Aciclovir, 200 mg five times daily for 5 days	• None required
Suppressive therapy (6–12 months)*		
• Aciclovir, 400 mg twice daily or 200 mg four times daily • Valaciclovir, 500 mg once daily • Famciclovir, 250 mg twice daily	• Seek expert advice	

*Antiviral therapy should be discontinued after 6–12 months' continuous use to reassess recurrence frequency.

Recurrent episode. Specific antiviral therapy is not usually required unless attacks are prolonged and/or frequent. Saline washes and simple analgesics can be recommended.

Frequent/prolonged recurrent episodes. Patients experiencing six or more episodes in a year and/or less frequent but prolonged bouts (lasting longer than 4 days) may benefit from a period of suppressive therapy (Table 10.1), the aim being to prevent recurrence.

Pregnancy. Most neonatal herpes (up to 70%) occurs in infants whose mothers do not have a history of genital herpes. In women who develop clinical episodes in pregnancy, management depends on whether the attack is recurrent or primary.

Recurrent herpes. Clinical recurrences in the first and second trimesters are unlikely to have any sequelae. If a recurrence occurs at or near delivery, the risk of neonatal infection is 1–4% (i.e. very low). If active lesions are present at the time of delivery, a cesarean section is often recommended, though it is not proven that this reduces the risk of transmission. If recommended, it should be performed within 4–6 hours of membrane rupture. Women with a history of herpes can have routine antenatal care. If troublesome recurrences occur during the pregnancy, expert advice about treatment options should be sought.

Primary herpes in early pregnancy. The most common outcomes of a primary attack are either miscarriage or an unaffected fetus. Primary herpes in the third trimester is associated with a risk of neonatal transmission of up to 50%. Urgent expert advice should be sought if primary herpes is diagnosed in pregnancy.

Prevention of neonatal infection. Neonatal herpes is often a catastrophic condition that can result in severe illness, disability and death. Of all cases, 35–50% relate to primary infection in pregnancy, the remaining cases relating to reactivation at or around delivery. Prevention therefore involves avoidance of primary infection and identification of the risk of recurrent herpes. A careful antenatal assessment, checking for a history of herpes in the woman and/or her partner, together with an assessment of current sexual risk, is important. Condom use and/or avoidance of intercourse towards term may be recommended if a risk is identified.

Follow-up. An individual diagnosed with primary herpes should be reviewed to ensure that the symptoms have settled without complications, to provide further information regarding the nature of the infection and to offer full STI screening for concurrent infections (see Table 2.4, page 17).

Contact tracing/partner notification. HSV is often passed within stable relationships by an asymptomatic carrier or an undiagnosed index case. The rate of transmission is 8–11% per year. It is useful to see partners to explain the diagnosis and discuss asymptomatic carriage and transmission. Given the opportunity to discuss the range of presenting symptoms, up to 50% of apparently asymptomatic carriers will give a history suggestive of one or more episodes of genital herpes.

External genital warts

There are more than 90 types of human papillomavirus (HPV) but approximately 30 types are associated with genital infection. The types that commonly cause genital warts are types 6 and 11, which are usually referred to as low-risk HPV types, indicative of their low or absent oncogenic potential.

Transmission. HPV is passed through close physical (skin-to-skin) contact. The incubation period is difficult to determine precisely, but the minimum period is probably 1 month. Some patients develop warts months, or even years, after initial exposure. Immunocompromised patients and pregnant women may develop warts after carrying the virus subclinically for months or years. In addition, only a proportion of infected patients will develop macroscopic genital warts; a substantial amount of transmission occurs as a result of subclinical infection.

Clinical features. Symptoms in both sexes include genital growths, which may:

- be hard or soft, and range from solitary (Figure 10.4a) to multiple
- bleed, particularly if meatal warts are present
- itch occasionally
- be pigmented.

In men, warts are commonly found on the penis (Figure 10.4b) and/or the urethra (careful examination of the urethra immediately proximal to the meatus is important in all patients), the perianal region (this is not exclusive to homosexual and bisexual men) and, rarely, on the scrotum. In women, warts are found on the vulva (Figure 10.4a), perianal area, cervix (Figure 10.4c), vagina (less commonly) and, infrequently, the urethra.

Complications and associations. The most important complication of some genital HPV types is genital epithelial cancer. External genital

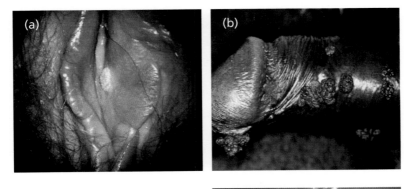

Figure 10.4 Genital warts: (a) solitary vulval wart; (b) penile shaft warts; (c) exophytic cervical wart and flat human papillomavirus change after application of 5% acetic acid.

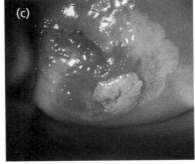

warts are most commonly caused by HPV 6 and 11, which are rarely associated with severe dysplasia and do not cause genital or anal cancers. However HPV 16, 18, 31, 33 and several other genital strains are oncogenic. There is an increased risk of cervical cancer and other genital tract neoplasia in infected patients, particularly those with persistent infection (> 12 months) with oncogenic subtypes. Genital warts may be associated with abnormal cervical smears. In the past, more frequent cervical smear (Pap) tests have been recommended for women with external genital warts, but guidance is now changing and local cervical screening policies should be followed. Tests for the detection of oncogenic HPV types are becoming available. They have a role in cervical screening, particularly in women with persistent low-grade abnormalities and in women over 30 years of age, where the positive predictive value of the tests goes up significantly. Genital warts and dysplasia are more pronounced in patients with immunodeficiency, for example in HIV infection or in iatrogenic immunodeficiency, such as that following renal transplantation.

Diagnosis is usually clinical and is based on the characteristic appearance of genital warts. Visual examination under good light, which may be aided by a magnifying glass, is the only recommended method for routine diagnosis. There is no place for HPV typing in routine clinical practice. Patients with external genital warts do not generally have any associated symptoms apart from occasional itching, and usually present because they have noticed or felt growths. Sometimes contact tracing will identify patients with previously unrecognized warts. A biopsy should be taken if there is any doubt about the diagnosis (e.g. if there is pigmentation, ulceration or other atypical characteristics). Up to 20% of patients presenting with first-episode genital warts have other STIs. Full screening for STIs is therefore recommended.

Treatment. Anogenital warts are essentially a cosmetic problem but often cause patients considerable psychological and psychosexual distress. The aim of treatment is to eradicate visible warts by destroying affected tissue (Table 10.2). Currently available therapies do not guarantee eradication of the virus. It is important to explain to patients that they may remain infectious even in the absence of visible warts. Recent studies, however, suggest that the majority of patients clear virus within 12 months of acquisition.

Prevention. New vaccines for preventing HPV infection have been approved for use in Europe and the USA in women and girls aged 9–26 years. Ideally, women should be vaccinated before their first sexual experience. Most public health infectious disease authorities also recommend vaccination for men. Some of the HPV vaccine formulations also include protection against HPV 6 and 11, which are the predominant causes of genital warts.

Pregnancy. Warts may present in pregnancy for the first time but may be more difficult to treat at this time. Certain topical therapies are contraindicated in pregnancy (Table 10.2). However, it is worth treating warts because some women do respond and the majority prefer not to have warts at the time of delivery. The risk of vertical transmission

TABLE 10.2

Treatment guidelines for external genital warts

Recommended regimens

- Podophyllotoxin, 0.5% solution or 0.15% cream, applied twice daily for 3 days, followed by a 4-day rest interval, then applied to lesions at weekly intervals
- Cryotherapy using a freeze–thaw–freeze cycle, at once- or twice-weekly intervals
- Podophyllin 15–25% solution, applied to lesions at once- or twice-weekly intervals; the solution should be washed off after 4 hours
- Trichloroacetic acid solution (80–90%)

Alternative regimens

- Electrocautery
- Imiquimod cream, applied three times a week at night until lesions resolve, for a maximum of 16 weeks

Regimen in pregnancy

- Cryotherapy using a freeze–thaw–freeze cycle, at once- or twice-weekly intervals
- Trichloroacetic acid solution (80–90%)
- Electrocautery

Contact treatment

- Only if warts present, then as recommended regimens

appears to be very low, but this view is controversial. On the basis of current evidence, the presence of genital warts should not influence the management of delivery. However, some experts recommend cesarean section to avoid laryngeal papillomatosis in the baby.

Follow-up. Patients should be monitored during treatment to check for efficacy and non-response (in which case treatment should be changed). Recurrence rates are high, and multiple rounds of treatment may be required.

Contact tracing/partner notification. Up to 60% of the contacts of patients with first-episode genital warts will also have warts. Known contacts who do not have any exophytic genital warts should be advised about self-examination of the genitals and that most persons who develop warts as a result of recent contact do so within several months. The current local policies for cervical smear recall should be followed for all female HPV contacts.

Molluscum contagiosum

The causative agent is a poxvirus.

Transmission occurs as a result of close physical contact, both sexual and non-sexual.

Complications. There are no significant complications in the immunocompetent host, and the virus causes a self-limiting infection. In immunocompromised patients (e.g. HIV-positive patients), lesions may be seen in atypical sites, such as the face and neck (see Figure 11.1), can be unusually large (giant molluscum) and may respond poorly to treatment.

Clinical features. Diagnosis is made on the basis of the highly characteristic appearance of an umbilicated pearly lesion, usually less than 2 mm diameter. Molluscum may be found on genital (Figure 10.5) and non-genital skin (see Figure 11.1).

Pregnancy. Molluscum contagiosum diagnosed in pregnancy does not pose any special risk. Cryotherapy can be used safely.

Treatment guidelines are summarized in Table 10.3.

Contact tracing/partner treatment. Contacts of patients with molluscum contagiosum can be seen and treated. Asymptomatic contacts do not need to be treated.

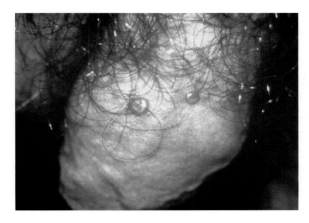

Figure 10.5
Molluscum
contagiosum on
the penile shaft.

TABLE 10.3

Treatment guidelines for molluscum contagiosum*

Recommended regimens

- Cryotherapy
- Expression of the pearly core, either manually or using forceps
- Piercing with an orange stick, with or without the application of tincture of iodine or phenol
- Curettage or diathermy under local anesthesia
- Podophyllotoxin 0.5% cream

Regimen in pregnancy

- Cryotherapy and other purely mechanical methods of destruction are safe
- Podophyllotoxin should not be used

Contact treatment

- None required unless lesions present, then as recommended regimens

*The natural history is spontaneous regression of lesions; treatment is offered for cosmetic reasons only.

Key points – herpes simplex, human papillomavirus infections and molluscum contagiosum

Herpes simplex virus
- Herpes can be transmitted only when an infected individual is shedding virus, which can occur both asymptomatically and when lesions are present.
- The clinical presentation is variable. A minority, probably fewer than 25%, will develop a severe primary attack.
- Recurrent episodes are often mild and infrequent.

External genital warts
- Not all infected patients develop macroscopic genital warts; a substantial proportion of transmission occurs from subclinical infection.
- The diagnosis is usually clinical and based on the characteristic appearance of genital warts.
- Anogenital warts are essentially a cosmetic problem, but often cause considerable psychological and psychosexual distress.
- The aim of treatment is to eradicate visible warts by destroying affected tissue; eradication of the virus is not guaranteed.
- Patients may remain infectious even in the absence of visible warts; however, the majority probably clear the virus within 12 months of infection.

Molluscum contagiosum
- The causative virus is transmitted by sexual and non-sexual contact.
- Infection is self-limiting, except in immunocompromised patients.

Blood-borne viruses: hepatitis B and C, HIV and AIDS

Hepatitis B

The hepatitis B virus (HBV) is a hepadnavirus (a small DNA virus).

Transmission. HBV is transmitted sexually, vertically and through contaminated blood products, either in a healthcare setting or during intravenous substance misuse. HBV is about ten times more infectious than human immunodeficiency virus (HIV). There are two carrier states:

- the highly infectious super-carrier state in which the hepatitis B 'e' antigen (HBeAg) is expressed
- the much less infectious hepatitis B surface 's' antigen (HBsAg) carrier.

Intravenous drug users and homosexual/bisexual men have high rates of infection with HBV, with 30–40% showing serological evidence of past infection.

Clinical features. Hepatitis B can cause acute infection of the liver that may manifest as an icteric illness or may be detected incidentally as raised transaminase levels, but 60–80% of patients acquire HBV infection silently and are diagnosed only in retrospect on serological screening. Women tend to have more severe disease than men. Hepatitis B can persist as a chronic infection (> 6 months).

Complications. Fewer than 1% of patients with acute infectious hepatitis will develop fulminant hepatic failure. Chronic infection will develop in 5–10%, with 20–30% of this group developing cirrhosis or carcinoma of the liver as a consequence of HBV infection. HBeAg-positive carriers have a higher risk of developing complications. A HIV-positive patient who acquires hepatitis B has an 18–20% chance of becoming a chronic carrier.

Diagnosis is made on serology (Table 11.1). In acute infection, blood tests are repeated over time to monitor liver dysfunction and to look for the development of antibodies. In asymptomatic disease, serology may indicate natural immunity or detect HBeAg and/or HBsAg. For people who are found to be antigen-positive at initial screening, repeat testing is recommended at, or after, 6 months to establish whether it is a recent acute infection, in which case the patient may develop immunity with time, or reflects an established carrier status.

Prevention. Hepatitis B is an STI that is almost completely preventable through immunization. Furthermore, the World Health Organization has recommended that HBV vaccine be incorporated into national immunization programs, regardless of prevalence. Many countries, including the USA, now have a universal program of infant vaccination. Where universal vaccination does not take place, 'at-risk' groups should be screened and immunized before exposure to infection. High-risk groups include:
- homosexual and bisexual men
- commercial sex workers
- heterosexuals with multiple sexual partners
- intravenous drug users and their contacts.

For patients who present acutely after recent exposure to a definite carrier, a combination of immunoglobulin and immediate vaccination may prevent infection. Victims of rape or sexual assault may benefit from immediate immunization – a risk assessment should be performed.

Treatment. Patients who present with acute hepatitis B in the primary care setting can be monitored and usually do not require hospital admission. Patients who develop 'e' antibodies but remain HBsAg-positive require annual liver function tests; referral should be considered if an abnormality develops. Patients with chronic infection and persistent HBeAg carriers should be referred to a specialist.

Pregnancy. Acute hepatitis B is associated with an increased rate of miscarriage/premature labor and in the third trimester is associated with a risk of transmission of up to 90%. The risk of perinatal

TABLE 11.1

Interpretation of hepatitis B serology

Stage of infection	HBsAg	HBeAg	IgM anticore antibody	IgG anticore antibody	Anti-HBe	Anti-HBs
Acute (early)	+	+	+	+	–	–
Acute (resolving)	+	–	+	+	+/–	–
Chronic (high infectivity)	+	+	–	+	–	–
or						
	+	–	–	+	–	–
Chronic (low infectivity)	+	–	–	+	+/–	–
Resolved (immune)	–	–	–	+	+/–	+/–
Successful vaccination	–	–	–	–	–	> 100 IU/L

HBsAg, hepatitis B surface 's' antigen; HBeAg, hepatitis B 'e' antigen; Ig, immunoglobulin.

transmission is up to 20% in HBsAg carriers and up to 50% for HBeAg carriers. Almost all babies who acquire HBV become carriers, and the risk of serious hepatic sequelae in later life is much higher among those who become infected during infancy/early childhood. Thus, all babies born to women who are HBV carriers should receive passive and active immunization at birth. Non-immune pregnant women exposed to HBV can be given passive and active immunization.

Contact tracing/partner notification. Contacts of hepatitis carriers (HBsAg and/or HBeAg positive) should be screened for HBV. HBV-negative contacts should be immunized. If there is an acute exposure to a known case of infectious hepatitis B, postexposure prophylaxis with vaccine should be offered as soon as possible (if less than 6 weeks after exposure) to the carrier. HBV-specific immunoglobulin should only be given within 72 hours of first exposure.

Hepatitis C

Hepatitis C virus (HCV) is endemic worldwide, with high prevalence in south and east Asia, north Africa and eastern Europe. UK prevalence varies from 0.06% in blood donors to 40% in intravenous drug users.

Transmission. In most cases HCV is acquired parenterally through shared needles/syringes in intravenous drug users, renal dialysis or needle-stick injury. Before the 1990s, it was also acquired through transfusion of infected blood or blood products. Amongst blood donors, 50% of those with HCV infection do not admit to having risk factors. A minority of cases of hepatitis C (< 5%) result from sexual or vertical transmission. The rate of seroconversion after unprotected vaginal or anal sex is about 2% per year if neither partner is infected with HIV, but the risk rises to over 10% if either partner is HIV-positive.

Clinical features. Infection is usually acquired asymptomatically. Hepatic illness develops in 5–10% of patients but is generally mild. In some studies, up to half of acute infections cleared spontaneously without treatment.

Complications. Studies suggest that the majority (60–70%) of infected individuals develop chronic infection. As with HBV infection, 15–30% will develop cirrhosis, with an increased risk of liver cancer over the next 10–50 years. Patients with concomitant liver disease or HIV infection or who drink alcohol at all are at increased risk for complications.

Diagnosis is based on the detection of antibodies, which develop about 3 months after infection. All patients found to have detectable HCV antibodies on screening should be tested for HCV RNA to confirm persistent viral replication. Diagnostic tests for HCV are recommended for the following:
- anyone presenting with suspected acute hepatitis
- patients with symptoms or signs of chronic liver disease or abnormal liver function tests consistent with acute or chronic hepatitis
- patients with any history (current or remote) of intravenous drug use.

Seroconversion may take 3 months, so antibody tests may give negative results when a patient presents with acute hepatitis. HCV RNA can be detected as early as 2 weeks after infection, so detection of HCV RNA by reverse transcriptase polymerase chain reaction (RT-PCR) will establish or exclude the diagnosis at this time. Detection of HCV RNA should be repeated 6 months after an episode of acute hepatitis C to confirm whether the infection has become chronic.

Prevention. Most HCV is acquired parenterally as a result of intravenous drug use, through the sharing of contaminated equipment to prepare or inject drugs. The use of clean needles will thus reduce transmission drastically. Sexual transmission is low in the absence of HIV coinfection, although HCV carriers should be encouraged to use barrier methods of protection. In long-term, stable relationships where childbearing is desired, couples may decide not to use a barrier method and to accept the very low risk of seroconversion.

Treatment. The recommended treatment for moderate-to-severe hepatitis C is 6 months' combination therapy using interferon-alpha and ribavarin, which has an efficacy of approximately 50%. Treatment is best provided in specialist centers.

Pregnancy. Data on hepatitis C during pregnancy are limited. The risk of vertical transmission is low (< 5%) and only women with detectable HCV RNA appear to be at risk of transmitting the infection; coinfection with HIV appears to increase the risk (up to 40%).

HIV/AIDS
HIV types I and II (retroviruses) are responsible for HIV infection and acquired immune deficiency syndrome (AIDS).

Transmission is sexual in 90% of adult infections worldwide. It also occurs vertically and through contaminated blood or blood products either in a healthcare context, particularly in the developing world, or from needle sharing during substance abuse.

Clinical features. HIV infection causes a disease spectrum in which patients progress from seroconversion, through asymptomatic infection to the diagnosis of AIDS. Primary HIV infection is commonly asymptomatic, but, on close questioning, up to 50% of patients report a self-limiting acute, mononucleosis-like illness within 3 months of acquiring infection. Primary infection is associated with acute immunodeficiency, and some patients may present with infections more characteristically associated with late HIV infection and AIDS, such as oral candidiasis and *Pneumocystis jirovecii* (*P. carinii*) pneumonia. A high index of suspicion will help in making the diagnosis at this stage.

During early infection, the majority of HIV-infected individuals remain well – but infectious – for many years, with no symptoms or signs. Diagnosis depends on the identification of risk factors and/or HIV screening, for example during antenatal programs or blood donation.

HIV infection causes a gradual depletion of CD4 cells, which eventually puts the patient at risk of certain opportunistic infections and tumors. The risk of progression can be predicted using a combination of quantitative viral load assessment and CD4 count. The first indications of immune deterioration may be quite subtle, with diseases that may also occur in the immunocompetent, such as:

- chronic skin problems (dry skin/seborrheic dermatitis/psoriasis, either an exacerbation or developing for the first time)
- oral candidiasis, which is usually recurrent in HIV-positive patients
- molluscum contagiosum, which is usually atypical in some way (e.g. giant lesions or an atypical site, such as the face; Figure 11.1)
- shingles (herpes zoster), which may be multidermatomal
- fevers
- persistent generalized lymphadenopathy
- oral hairy leukoplakia (Figure 11.2).

In some patients, presentation may be with clinical syndromes associated with HIV infection (Table 11.2), including the more common HIV presentations of tuberculosis, Kaposi's sarcoma (Figure 11.3) and cytomegalovirus retinitis (Figure 11.4).

Diagnosis is based on the detection of anti-HIV antibodies. Antibodies are detectable in almost all infected patients if measured at least 3 months after exposure. An earlier diagnosis may be made using PCR.

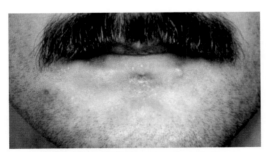

Figure 11.1 Facial molluscum contagiosum in an HIV-positive man.

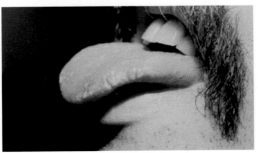

Figure 11.2 Oral hairy leukoplakia on the lateral border of the tongue in a patient infected with HIV.

TABLE 11.2

When to consider human immunodeficiency virus (HIV) infection in clinical practice: common syndromes associated with HIV

Diagnostic category	Clinical syndrome
Acute/early HIV infection	• Unexplained mononucleosis-like or viral illness in patient with risk factors for HIV
Symptomatic HIV infection (not AIDS): relative preservation of CD4 count > 0.2 × 10^9/L	• Recurrent oral candidiasis • Persistent generalized lymphadenopathy • Unexplained persistent thrombocytopenia • Seborrheic dermatitis – developing for the first time or increasingly severe existing disease • Atypical/giant molluscum (often facial) • White plaques on the lateral border of the tongue (oral hairy leukoplakia: see Figure 11.2)
Late symptomatic HIV infection/AIDS: CD4 count usually < 200*	• Pneumonia – usually atypical organisms, commonly *Pneumocystis jirovecii* (*P. carinii*) • Sore mouth and dysphagia – oro–esophageal candidiasis • Visual blurring/loss – cytomegalovirus disease • Neurological syndromes – space-occupying lesions (e.g. cerebral toxoplasmosis and cerebral lymphoma) • Skin lesions – Kaposi's sarcoma (CD4 count may be > 200)

*Some patients do not present for testing and may therefore be seen with a severe manifestation of late immunodeficiency.
AIDS, acquired immune deficiency syndrome.

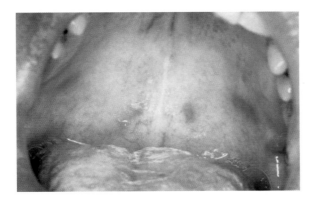

Figure 11.3
Kaposi's sarcoma
in the mouth.

Prevention. Consistent use of condoms is the main way of preventing the sexual transmission/acquisition of HIV. Targeting advice at high-risk groups may also be beneficial, and should include specific advice about safer sex practices for men who have sex with men (ideally avoidance of anal intercourse, even with the use of condoms and lubrication), as well as methods for reducing the risks for intravenous drug users.

Pregnancy. The risk of vertical transmission can be reduced to approximately 2% using a combination of antiretroviral drugs, elective cesarean section and avoiding breastfeeding. Prevention of vertical transmission depends on the identification and screening of

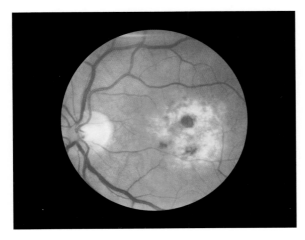

Figure 11.4
Cytomegalovirus
retinitis in a
patient with
acquired immune
deficiency
syndrome.

high-risk women. In the UK, universal screening is now part of routine antenatal care. (Selective screening did not prove effective in identifying women at risk.)

Treatment. Highly active antiretroviral treatment (HAART; usually a combination of three or more drugs) and the use of prophylactic antibiotics to prevent opportunistic infections are the mainstay of treatment. Drug therapy for HIV/AIDS is complicated and beyond the scope of this text. HIV-infected patients should be monitored regularly in centers with the appropriate expertise.

Contact tracing/partner notification can be particularly difficult, as patients may have been infected for months or years before diagnosis. Ideally, all traceable partners should be seen and counseled with a view to testing.

Key points – blood-borne viruses: hepatitis B and C and HIV/AIDS

Hepatitis B virus (HBV)
- 60–80% of patients acquire HBV silently and are diagnosed only in retrospect on serological screening.
- 5–10% of infected individuals will develop chronic infection, and 20–30% of this group develop cirrhosis or carcinoma of the liver.
- HBV is almost completely preventable through immunization.

Hepatitis C virus (HCV)
- In most cases HCV is acquired parenterally through shared needles/syringes in intravenous drug users, through transfusion of blood or blood products (pre-1990s), renal dialysis or needle-stick injury.
- Infection is usually acquired asymptomatically.
- The majority (60–70%) of infected individuals develop chronic infection: 15–30% will develop cirrhosis with an increased risk of liver cancer over the next 10–50 years.

HIV/AIDS
- HIV infection causes a disease spectrum in which patients may progress from seroconversion, through asymptomatic infection, to a diagnosis of AIDS.
- Following infection, the majority of HIV-infected individuals remain well with no symptoms or signs for many years, but are nevertheless infectious.
- Diagnosis depends on the identification of risk factors and/or HIV screening and is based on the detection of HIV antibodies.
- HIV infection causes depletion of CD4 cells, which eventually puts the patient at risk of opportunistic infections and tumors.

Trichomonas vaginalis

T. vaginalis is a flagellated protozoon.

Transmission. In adults, *T. vaginalis* is almost exclusively transmitted sexually; infection follows intravaginal or intraurethral inoculation of the organism. Opinions vary as to whether *T. vaginalis* can be transmitted by non-sexual contact.

Clinical features. The symptoms and signs of trichomoniasis are described in Table 12.1. In women, the organism is found in the vagina and urethra. While the urinary tract is the sole site of infection in fewer than 5% of cases, urethral infection is present in 90%. In men, infection is usually of the urethra, although trichomonads have been isolated from the subpreputial sac and from lesions of the penis.

Examination of the male is usually normal, though there may be signs of urethritis. Women may have vulvitis, vaginitis and excessive

TABLE 12.1

Symptoms and signs of trichomoniasis

Women

- Asymptomatic (50%)
- Vaginal discharge (offensive, yellow, thin, frothy)
- Vulval irritation
- Superficial dyspareunia
- Dysuria (rare)

Men

- Usually asymptomatic (50–80%)
- Urethritis (20–50%)
- Balanitis (rare)

vaginal discharge (affecting up to 70%), which is characteristically yellow. The cervix may have the classic strawberry appearance (Figure 12.1), detectable without magnification in only a few but by colposcopy in up to 50%.

Complications. Recent evidence suggests that trichomoniasis is associated with adverse pregnancy outcome (see Pregnancy, below) and facilitates the sexual transmission of human immunodeficiency virus (HIV). However, these associations need to be confirmed and a causal association proved.

Diagnosis. Microscopy of a wet-mount preparation is the most commonly used diagnostic test for *T. vaginalis* infection. Characteristic motile, flagellated protozoa are readily seen. Microscopy for *T. vaginalis* should be performed as soon as possible after the sample is taken, as motility diminishes with time. A wet smear and/or acridine-orange slide from the posterior vaginal fornix will diagnose 40–80% of cases in women. Culture will diagnose up to 95% of cases. Trichomonads are sometimes reported on cervical cytology; sensitivity is approximately 60% but there is a high false-positive rate and it is prudent to confirm the diagnosis with a vaginal swab in such cases.

Diagnosis is much more difficult in men. Most are completely asymptomatic and, as a result, male partners of female patients should

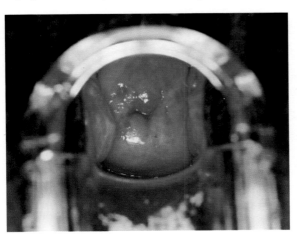

Figure 12.1
Strawberry cervix caused by trichomoniasis.

always be treated. A wet preparation from the urethra reveals infection in about 30% of cases. Urethral culture will diagnose 60–80% of cases.

Currently, culture techniques are still regarded as the most sensitive and specific. Several protocols have been described for the detection of *T. vaginalis* DNA using the polymerase chain reaction (PCR), but PCR assays for *T. vaginalis* are not yet commercially available.

Treatment. Because of the high rate of infection of the urethra and paraurethral glands in women, systemic chemotherapy should be given to provide a permanent cure. Most strains of *T. vaginalis* are highly susceptible to metronidazole and related drugs (see Table 12.2). Regular sexual partners should be treated simultaneously to maximize the cure rate. If this cannot be achieved, abstinence from sexual intercourse should be advised until the partner has been seen. Screening for coexisting STIs should be undertaken.

Pregnancy. *T. vaginalis* infection is associated with preterm delivery and low birth weight. Metronidazole can be used in all stages of pregnancy and during breastfeeding, although high-dose regimens are best avoided in these circumstances. However, recent trials have found that treatment

TABLE 12.2

Treatment guidelines for *Trichomonas vaginalis* infection

Recommended regimen
- Metronidazole, 400–500 mg twice daily for 5–7 days

Alternative regimens
- Metronidazole, 2 g as a single dose
- Tinidazole, 2 g as a single dose

Regimen in pregnancy
- Metronidazole, 400–500 mg twice daily for 5–7 days

Contact treatment
- Use recommended regimen

of *T. vaginalis* infection in pregnancy does not improve pregnancy outcome, and may be harmful; the best management, particularly of asymptomatic women, is therefore uncertain.

Follow-up. Tests of cure should be undertaken if the patient remains symptomatic after treatment or if symptoms recur.

Contact tracing/partner notification. Partners should be seen and treated regardless of test results. It is reasonable to treat a male contact with non-specific urethritis (NSU) for *T. vaginalis* initially, and then to repeat the urethral smear before making a diagnosis of NSU.

Pubic lice

The pubic louse, *Phthirus pubis*, is an ectoparasite that feeds on human blood. All five stages of the lifecycle occur on the human host. Infestation with *P. pubis* is also known as pediculosis.

Transmission. Human lice are transmitted from person to person by intimate contact; sexual transmission is the usual means of acquiring pubic lice.

Clinical features. The grasp of the pubic louse's claw matches that of the diameter and spacing of pubic and axillary hair. Lice may occasionally be found on the bearded area of the face, eyelashes and eyebrows. Head lice do not cause pubic infection.

The clinical presentation is related to allergic sensitization to the lice, and the main symptoms are scratching, erythema, irritation and inflammation. It takes a minimum of 5 days for this sensitization to develop. Both adult lice and nits (the eggs) attached to hairs can be seen by the naked eye. People infested for a long time may become oblivious to lice on their bodies. In some, however, excessive scratching leads to superinfection.

Diagnosis is based on clinical appearance (a magnifying glass may be useful), and can be confirmed by identifying the lice or nits using a low-powered microscope (Figure 12.2).

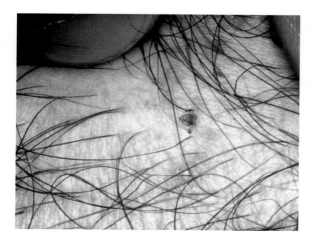

Figure 12.2
Pediculosis with classic hemorrhagic lesions.

Treatment. Topical treatment should be applied to all hairy areas except for the scalp, and washed off after 24 hours (Table 12.3). Occasionally a second treatment at 7–10 days will be necessary. Nits on the eyelashes

TABLE 12.3

Treatment guidelines for pubic lice

Recommended regimens

- Malathion 0.5%, applied to dry hair and washed out after at least 2 hours (preferably 12 hours)
- Permethrin 1% cream rinse, applied to damp hair and washed out after 10 minutes
- Phenothrin 0.2%, applied to dry hair and washed out after 2 hours
- Carbaryl 0.5% or 1%, applied to dry hair and washed out after 12 hours

Regimen in pregnancy

- Permethrin 1% cream rinse, applied to damp hair and washed out after 10 minutes

Contact treatment

- Use recommended regimens

should be combed out; application of petroleum jelly may be helpful. Other STIs should be sought and treated.

Pregnancy. No complications have been described. Gamma-benzene hexachloride (lindane) should not be used in pregnancy; it is lipid-soluble and can be excreted in breast milk.

Follow-up. Concurrent infections should be treated as appropriate, but follow-up of patients with *P. pubis* infestation is only necessary if symptoms persist.

Contact tracing/partner notification. Sexual partners and others in close bodily contact should also be screened for other STIs and treated.

Scabies
This condition is caused by the mite *Sarcoptes scabiei*.

Transmission results from fairly prolonged close physical contact, not necessarily sexual. Mites separated from the human host die after 72 hours.

Clinical features. Symptoms and signs arise 2–6 weeks after initial infestation, but may arise much more rapidly following reinfection. Symptoms result from sensitization to the mite. The most common complaint is itching that is usually worse at night or after a hot bath. A rash or papules may be noticed, particularly in the web spaces of the fingers or on the genitals, but also in the armpits or on the forearms, abdomen and buttocks (Figure 12.3).

Complications. A crusted form of scabies can occur in patients who are immunocompromised, including those infected with HIV. This may be widespread with a scaling appearance. The symptoms of itch are generally mild. Very rarely, a secondary streptococcal infection occurs, which may lead to acute glomerulonephritis.

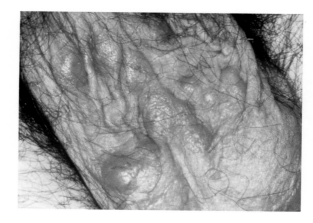

Figure 12.3
Scabies of the
scrotum and
ventral aspect of
the penis.

Diagnosis is based on the clinical history and examination, and can be confirmed by finding the mite. Scrape the top from the whole length of a burrow using a scalpel and examine for mites on a microscope slide with 10% potassium hydroxide.

Treatment. If acquisition of scabies is related to sexual contact, consider screening for other STIs. Topical treatment (Table 12.4) should be applied to the whole body from the neck downwards, and washed off after 12 hours – it is usually left on overnight. Potentially contaminated clothes and bedding should be washed at high temperature (above 50°C). It is important to understand that although symptoms of itch

---

TABLE 12.4

Treatment guidelines for scabies

Recommended regimens

- Permethrin 5% dermal cream (left on for 12 hours)
- Malathion 0.5% aqueous lotion (left on for 12 hours)

Regimen in pregnancy

- Permethrin 5% dermal cream (left on for 12 hours)

Contact treatment

- Use recommended regimens

may persist for several weeks, this does not reflect persistent infection. Antihistamines may provide symptomatic relief of itching.

Pregnancy. No complications have been described. Permethrin can be used during pregnancy and breastfeeding.

Follow-up. None is required unless symptoms persist or new lesions appear.

Contact tracing/partner notification. Sexual partners should be treated. If transmission was not sexual, household members and other close social contacts should be treated, even if asymptomatic.

Key points – trichomoniasis, pediculosis and scabies

Trichomoniasis
- In adults, *Trichomonas vaginalis* is almost exclusively sexually transmitted.
- The majority of infected men and women are asymptomatic.
- Regular sexual partners should be treated simultaneously to maximize the cure rate.
- Screening for coexisting STIs should be undertaken.

Pubic lice
- Sexual transmission is the usual means of acquiring pubic lice.
- Head lice do not cause pubic infestation.
- The clinical presentation of scratching, erythema, irritation and inflammation is related to allergic sensitization to the louse.

Scabies
- Transmission results from fairly prolonged close physical contact, not necessarily sexual.
- Symptoms proceed from sensitization to the mite.
- Symptoms of itch may persist for several weeks after effective treatment: this does not reflect persistent infection.

Useful resources

Websites

British Association for Sexual Health and HIV (UK)
National guidelines on sexually transmitted infections and related conditions
www.bashh.org/guidelines.asp
www.guideline.gov

Centers for Disease Control and Prevention (USA)
Morbidity and Mortality Weekly Report
www.cdc.gov/mmwr/

Centers for Disease Control and Prevention, Workowski KA, Berman SM. Clinical prevention guidance. Sexually transmitted diseases treatment guidelines 2006.
MMWR Recomm Rep 2006;55 (RR-11):1–94.
www.guideline.gov

Health Protection Agency (UK)
www.hpa.org.uk

HIV/AIDS treatment information service (USA)
www.hivatis.org

Johns Hopkins AIDS service (USA)
www.hopkins-aids.edu

National AIDS Manual (UK)
website with patient information and news on HIV/AIDS research and management
www.aidsmap.com

Royal College of General Practitioners (UK) and British Association for Sexual Health and HIV
Sexually transmitted infections in primary care 2006
www.bashh.org/primarycare/stis_primary_care_march2006.pdf

Organizations

American Sexually Transmitted Diseases Association
PO Box 133118
Atlanta, GA 30333-3118
Tel: +1 404 616 5606
Fax: +1 404 616 6847
http://depts.washington.edu/astda

American Social Health Association
PO Box 13827
Research Triangle Park, NC 27709
Tel: +1 919 361 8400
Fax: +1 919 361 8425
www.ashastd.org

British Association for Sexual Health and HIV
1 Wimpole Street
London W1G 0AE
Tel: +44 (0)20 7290 2968
Fax: +44 (0)20 7290 2989
bashh@rsm.ac.uk
www.bashh.org

European Surveillance of Sexually Transmitted Infections
Health Protection Agency
61 Colindale Avenue
London NW9 5EQ UK
Tel: +44 (0)20 8200 6868
Fax: +44 (0)20 8200 7868
essti@hpa.org.uk
www.essti.org

Genito-Urinary Nurses Association (UK)
www.guna.org.uk

Herpes Viruses Association (UK)
41 North Road
London N7 9DP
Tel: +44 (0)845 123 2305
info@herpes.org.uk
www.herpes.org.uk

International Union Against Sexually Transmitted Infections
Dr Raj Patel, IUSTI Secretary-General
The Royal South Hants Hospital
Brintons Terrace
Southampton SO14 OYG
Tel: +44 (23) 80 825152
Fax: +44 (23) 80 825122
www.iusti.org

Medical Foundation for Aids and Sexual Health (UK)
BMA House, Tavistock Square
London WC1H 9JP
Tel: +44 (0)20 8383 6345
Fax: +44 (0)870 442 1792
enquiries.medfash@medfash.bma.org.uk
www.medfash.org.uk

National Association of Nurses for Contraception & Sexual Health (UK)
9 Church Close, Drayton Bassett
Staffordshire B78 3UJ
Tel: +44 (0)1827 260117
Fax: +44 (0)1827 260154
info@nancsh.org.uk
www.nancsh.org.uk

National Coalition of STD Directors (USA)
1275 K Street NW, Suite 1000
Washington DC 20005
Tel: +1 202 842 4660
Fax: +1 202 842 4542
info@ncsddc.org
www.ncsddc.org

National Network of STD/HIV Prevention Training Centers (USA)
http://depts.washington.edu/nnptc/

Royal Australasian College of Physicians, Chapter of Sexual Health Medicine
145 Macquarie Street
Sydney NSW 2000
Tel: +61 (0)2 9256 9643
Fax: +61 (0)2 9256 9693
www.racp.edu.au/public/
sexualhealth.htm
sexualhealthmed@racp.edu.au

Society of Sexual Health Advisers (UK)
info@ssha.info
www.ssha.info

Terrence Higgins Trust (UK)
314–320 Gray's Inn Road
London WC1X 8DP
Tel: +44 (0)20 7812 1600
Fax: +44 (0)20 7812 1601
info@tht.org.uk
www.tht.org.uk

125

References

General

Holmes KK, Sparling PF, Mardh P-A et al., eds. *Sexually Transmitted Diseases*, 4th edn. New York: McGraw–Hill, 2006.

Centers for Disease Control and Prevention. Sexually Transmitted Disease Guidelines 2006. *Morbid Mortal Weekly Rep* 2006;55:RR11.

Sexually transmitted diseases. *Lancet* 1998;351(suppl 3):(entire issue).

Epidemiology and control

Centers for Disease Control and Prevention (USA). *2005 STD Surveillance Report.* www.cdc.gov/std/stats/default.htm

Collaborative Group for HIV and STI Surveillance (UK). *Mapping the Issues. HIV and Other Sexually Transmitted Infections in the United Kingdom: 2005.* London: Health Protection Agency Centre for Infections. November 2005. www.hpa.org.uk/publications/2005/hiv_sti_2005/pdf/MtI_FC_report.pdf

Communicable Disease Report Weekly (UK) www.hpa.org.uk/cdr/pages/hiv_STIs.htm

Johnson AM, Mercer CH, Erens B et al. Sexual behaviour in Britain: partnerships, practices, and HIV risk behaviours. *Lancet* 2001;358:1835–42.

Weinstock H, Berman S, Cates W Jr. Sexually transmitted diseases among American youth: incidence and prevalence estimates, 2000. *Persp Sex Reprod Health* 2004;36:6–10. www.guttmacher.org/pubs/journals/3600604.html

Approach to the patient

Holmes KK, Levine R, Weaver M. Effectiveness of condoms in preventing sexually transmitted infections. *Bull World Health Organ* 2004;82:454–61.

Pelvic inflammatory disease

Ross JDC. An update on pelvic inflammatory disease. *Sex Transm Infect* 2002;78:18–19.

Bacterial infections

Cook RL, Hutchison SL, Østergaard L et al. Systematic review: noninvasive testing for *Chlamydia trachomatis* and *Neisseria gonorrhoeae. Ann Intern Med* 2005;142:914–25.

Nelson HD, Helfand M. Screening for chlamydial infection. *Am J Prev Med* 2001;20:95–107.

Peipert JF. Genital chlamydial infections. *N Engl J Med* 2003;349:2424–30.

Rolfs RT, Joesoef MR, Hendershot EF et al. A randomized trial of enhanced therapy for early syphilis in patients with and without human immunodeficiency virus infection. *N Engl J Med* 1997;337:307–14.

Rompalo AM. Can syphilis be eradicated from the world? *Curr Opin Infect Dis* 2001;14:41–4.

US Preventive Services Task Force. Screening for chlamydial infection: recommendations and rationale. *Am J Prev Med* 2001;20:90–4.

Herpes simplex and human papillomavirus infections

Bundrick JB, Cook DA, Gostout BS. Screening for cervical cancer and initial treatment of patients with abnormal results from Papanicolaou testing. *Mayo Clin Proc* 2005;80:1063–8.

Burd EM. Human papillomavirus and cervical cancer. *Clin Microbiol Rev* 2003;16:1–17.

Corey L, Wald A, Patel R et al. Once-daily valacyclovir to reduce the risk of transmission of genital herpes. *N Engl J Med* 2004;350:11–20.

Kimberlin DW, Rouse DJ. Genital herpes. *N Engl J Med* 2004;350:1970–7.

Partridge JM, Koutsky LA. Genital human papillomavirus infection in men. *Lancet Infect Dis* 2006;6:21–31.

Sasieni P, Adams J, Cuzick J. Benefit of cervical screening at different ages: evidence from the UK audit of screening histories. *Br J Cancer* 2003;89:88–93.

Blood-borne viruses: hepatitis B and C and HIV/AIDS

Branson BM, Handsfield HH, Lampe MA et al. Revised recommendations for HIV testing of adults, adolescents, and pregnant women in health-care settings. *MMWR Recomm Rep* 2006;55:1–17.

Centers for Disease Control and Prevention. *HIV Prevention Case Management Guidance*. Atlanta, Georgia: Centers for Disease Control and Prevention, 1997. www.cdc.gov/hiv/topics/prev_prog/CRCS/resources/PCMG/index.htm

Trichomoniasis

Schwebke JR, Burgess D. Trichomoniasis. *Clin Microbiol Rev* 2004;17:794–803.

Index

129

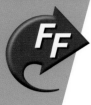
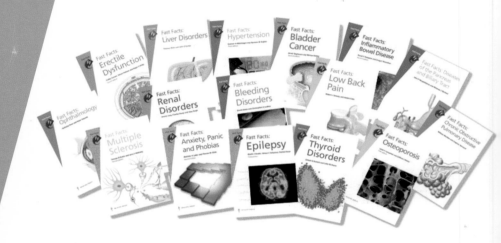